GET
THROUGH

DCH Clinical

GET THROUGH

DCH Clinical

Second Edition

Jasdeep Gill MB ChB (Hons) DRCOG DFSRH DCH
GP Registrar, London Deanery

Andrew Papanikitas BSc (Hons) MA MBBS DCH MRCGP
Portfolio GP, PhD Student, Department of
Education and Professional Studies and
Sessional Tutor, King's College London

Nigel Kennedy MBBS FRCP FRCPCH DCH DRCOG DTM & H
Retired GP and hospital practitioner
(Paediatrics), Aylesbury

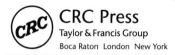

CRC Press
Taylor & Francis Group
Boca Raton   London   New York

CRC Press is an imprint of the
Taylor & Francis Group, an **informa** business

CRC Press
Taylor & Francis Group
6000 Broken Sound Parkway NW, Suite 300
Boca Raton, FL 33487-2742

**Library of Congress Cataloging-in-Publication Data and
The British Library Cataloging in Publication Data are Available**

**Visit the Taylor & Francis Web site at
http://www.taylorandfrancis.com**

**and the CRC Press Web site at
http://www.crcpress.com**

Printed and bound by CPI Group (UK) Ltd, Croydon, CR0 4YY

CONTENTS

ACKNOWLEDGEMENTS

With thanks to Hodder Education for their hard work and cooperation and to Dr Helen Goodliffe, who co-authored the first edition.

We dedicate this book to all upcoming doctors with an interest in paediatrics, and to our families.

FOREWORD

The responsibility for delivering Primary Child Health Care in the United Kingdom lies with general practitioners (GPs) and it is essential that they are adequately trained and experienced in looking after children. All GPs see children in routine surgeries every day and should have a good working knowledge of basic child health care. Possession of the DCH diploma is appropriate proof of that.

There is a trend towards some GPs developing a special interest in a specific clinical field such as paediatrics, orthopaedics, ENT, dermatology etc. Even if DCH is not taken up as an essential universal foundation qualification for GPs, it is important that GPs with a special interest in child care should have a method of demonstrating their competence as shown by passing the DCH.

Candidates who wish to take the DCH examination have to pass a written test of basic child health knowledge before they can progress to the clinical exam. Once they have done that, the most important part of training to get through the clinical examination is practical experience. Thus, it is essential that candidates prepare themselves by attending child health clinics in the community as well as in hospitals and practise medical examinations, including developmental assessment. While this 'in vivo' experience is crucial, there are several other methods of adding 'in vitro' training to increase the chances of passing the examination. There are several books available on the DCH examination but few devoted exclusively to the clinical component. This book, 'Get Through DCH Clinical' delivers 'what it says on the tin' and is a very good, up-to-date account of what candidates will be faced with on the day of the clinical exam and how to successfully manoeuvre their way through the stations.

The first chapter draws an accurate map of the examination structure and prepares the candidate for the obstacles that they will meet and how they are organised.

The next 7 chapters are each devoted to a single OSCE station and give detailed descriptions of format, approach and common themes of situations that the candidate will be presented with. The order of the chapters is arbitrary as each candidate will start the clinical cycle at a different station. However, the cycles are divided into the 'Talking' stations (communication/data interpretation/structured oral) and the 'Clinical' stations (clinical assessment/focused history/child development).

The description of each station tells readers everything that they need to know about what to expect. Examples of possible scenarios and situations are given with tips on how to approach and address examiners, role players and patients. These examples are worked through in considerable detail with appropriate answers. The 'Anchor statements', which are the formal guidelines given to examiners about how to apply Pass/Fail standards to a candidate's performance, are provided. It is very helpful to have these clearly attached to each station in the respective chapters.

The current DCH clinical examination places great importance on communication skills and the book clearly points out that a candidate must demonstrate a high level of competence in this area, not only in the Communication stations, but also in every other station in the cycle. The candidate must know how to deal with children plus their attached adults, in a sympathetic, sensitive and non-intimidating manner. One of the strengths of a multi-station examination is that candidates will meet several different examiners and they must be able to communicate effectively with each of them. This book gives clear advice on how to communicate with all the people that a candidate will meet during the course of the examination.

A further aspect of the DCH is that it is not 'rocket science' and a candidate who has a good understanding and factual knowledge about basic paediatrics and child health is well placed to attain a pass in DCH. Candidates who get bogged down in small print details but have difficulty prioritising more common events and problems are more likely to have difficulties. The examples given in each chapter give clear examples of appropriate answers which are quite sufficient.

Chapters 5 and 7 describe the stations where children will always be present and give very good advice on how the candidate should perform appropriate assessments, again with relevant examples.

A candidate who reads this book will be well prepared to face all situations that are likely to come up in the course of the DCH clinical examination. It should be regarded as an additional resource to practical teaching and experience for any candidate who wishes to maximise their chances of passing DCH.

Dr Martin Bellman
Consultant Paediatrician
Royal Free Hospital, London

PREFACE

The Diploma in Child Health (DCH) is an extremely useful qualification. Paediatrics forms a significant proportion of daily consultations in general practice and of the RCGP core curriculum. We recommend undertaking the DCH to all GPs and GP trainees to enhance your paediatric knowledge and skills for community practice.

This book is a revision aid to help you prepare for the DCH clinical examination. It includes a wide range of clinical scenarios and cases for you to practise. GP trainees may also find this book and preparation for the DCH examination helpful when preparing for the clinical skills assessment for the MRCGP.

We hope that this book will help you prepare for the exam and understand that children are not little adults, but they are not little terrors either!

Best of luck.

Jasdeep Gill
Andrew Papanikitas
Nigel Kennedy

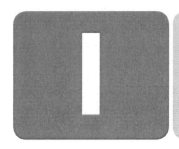

INTRODUCTION

Paediatrics forms a significant proportion of daily consultations in general practice, with almost 30% of an average general practice population comprising of children. A holistic approach to child health is essential, because general practitioners (GPs) are not only responsible for the acute and chronic conditions, but also child development, health promotion, screening programmes and child protection. GPs must be able to work with the numerous agencies now involved in the multidisciplinary approach to childcare and to recognize when to seek assistance from the appropriate agency.

The DCH examination

This diploma assesses all spheres of paediatric care and passing the diploma demonstrates that the doctor has achieved the appropriate level of competency to carry out their responsibilities to children. It is geared towards GPs or GP trainees, and the scenarios generally refer to the candidate as a GP.

The DCH examination is set by the Royal College of Paediatrics and Child Health and consists of two parts: Part 1 is a multiple choice paper called the MRCPCH Part 1A, which consists of multiple true/false questions, best of five questions and extended matching questions. Upon satisfactory completion of this, DCH candidates then undertake the second part of the assessment: the DCH Clinical Examination, which from 2006 has been conducted as an OSCE (Objective Structured Clinical Examination) held at centres across England and Wales. DCH candidates may sit the DCH Clinical (Part 2) on three occasions only and if unsuccessful are then required to resit Part 1 again.

DCH Clinical examination

The DCH Clinical examination consists of eight OSCE stations. These eight stations are divided into two circuits (Figure 1.1). Circuit A will last 36 minutes in total, with each station lasting 6 minutes and 3-minute intervals between each station. Circuit B will last a total of 48 minutes, with each station lasting 9 minutes and 3-minute intervals between each station. Each candidate's sequence of stations will vary depending on the station at which the candidate starts.

Each circuit has two 'cycles' of candidates (i.e. two sets of circuit A will run at the same time). As the candidate, you will move from one station to the next. The examiner will remain in the same station for that cycle. There will be a 40-minute

Circuit A: 6-minute stations

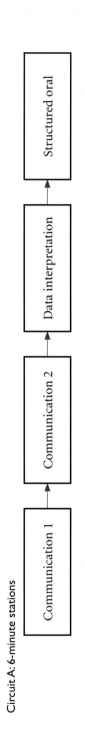

Circuit B: 9-minute stations

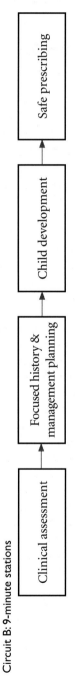

Figure 1.1 DCH OSCE cycle.

break between the circuits. This allows the examiners and role players or patients to reorganize themselves and prepare for the next circuit.

There will be 12 objective assessments made of each candidate during the entire eight stations. The circuit A (6-minute) stations carry 1 assessment each and the circuit B (9-minute) stations carry two assessments each – giving a total of 12 assessments.

How to prepare for the DCH Clinical

Start your preparation early. As with all clinical examinations, you will learn and hone your skills over time. The DCH Clinical is certainly not something you can cram for overnight. Having a clear understanding of the OSCE format (Figure 1.1) will help you focus your revision. You should also visit the Royal College of Paediatrics and Child Health (RCPCH) website (http://www.rcpch.ac.uk/ Examinations/DCH), which has useful information about the syllabus to help you identify gaps in your knowledge.

Spend as much time as possible seeing and examining children. This can be in general or specialist paediatric clinics, GP surgeries or on the wards. Be innovative when not at work, for example, do developmental 'checks' on babies or children you see while out or ask family and friends if you can practise an examination on their child. Examining babies and children with no pathology is vitally important for you to establish an understanding of normal, and be aware that children with no pathology are often recruited for clinical examinations. *Make sure that you obtain consent from parents or if appropriate the child before conducting any practise examination.*

The RCPCH will send you candidate instructions well in advance of the examination. Make sure you read these very carefully and fully digest the information. Not only does this pack include vital information about the date, time and venue of your examination, but it also includes helpful resource documents about the examination.

Make sure you get the logistical aspects in order. Don't forget to arrange for leave on the day of your examination. Always plan your journey well in advance and account for traffic, public transport strikes or natural disasters! It may be worthwhile staying in a nearby hotel to help alleviate some stress on the day.

Remember to take certain items with you on the day of the examination. You must have your candidate invitation letter with you which has your unique RCPCH identification number on it. A proof of identification is required. This must be a photographic form of identification, so either your driving license or passport. You are likely to need a stethoscope for the clinical station. Don't worry if you do not have a paediatric stethoscope, but make sure you are comfortable using whichever stethoscope you have. Most other clinical equipment is provided if needed.

> ## Checklist of things to remember
> ✓ Candidate letter and ID number
> ✓ Photographic proof of identification
> ✓ Stethoscope
> ✓ Pen torch
> ✓ Disposable measuring tap
> ✓ Small (cleanable) toy
> ✓ Food and drink

A pen torch and measuring tape may be helpful to have in your pocket to help conserve valuable seconds in case they are needed. Most candidates take a small toy with them, which is often not required but can sometimes be helpful to distract or pacify a child. You must ensure, however, that the toy is safe to use, with no dangerous or small parts, and it should be cleaned in between uses by patients. Finally, not all examination centres provide refreshments for candidates, so you should take some food and drink with you.

What to expect on the day

Expect to be nervous! Do not be put off by your nerves or by other candidates around you who seem to be exuding confidence and knowledge. Some candidates are chatty, even when nervous, while others prefer to be left alone to cram in as many last-minute revision topics as they can. Take a moment to consider how you will spend the time before your exam to help optimize your performance. You should aim to be composed and confident, but do not appear arrogant.

Most examination centres will take a photograph of you. This is to help the examiners recall each candidate clearly when debriefing at the end of the day.

You will be told which station to start on and you will cycle onwards from there. Make sure you use the intervals between each station wisely! Use this time to forget about the station before and compose yourself for the next station. If there is a brief available for your next station, read it thoroughly and consider how you will tackle the scenario and things you want to cover within the short timeframe of the station. Tables 1.1 and 1.2 should help you visualize and understand how the total circuit time will be used.

Table 1.1 Circuit A timeframe

Station	Reading (during interval)	6-minute assessment	Warning sound
Communication 1	Read scenario outside room (approx. 2 min)	Assessment with role player and examiner	Given when 1 min remaining
Communication 2	Read scenario outside room (approx. 2 min)	Assessment with role player and examiner	Given when 1 min remaining
Data interpretation	No data sheet available until room entered	2 min: interpret data 4 min: discuss with examiner	Given when 1 min remaining
Structured oral	No details available until room entered	1–2 min: read scenario 4–5 min: discuss with examiner	Given when 1 min remaining

Table 1.2 Circuit B timeframe

Station	Reading (during interval)	9-minute assessment	Warning sound
Clinical assessment	No details available until room entered	Assessment with role player and examiner	Given when 1 min remaining
Focused history/ management	Read scenario outside room (approx. 2 min)	6 min: history with role player. Role player leaves. 3 min: discuss with examiner	Given when 4 min remaining
Child development	No data sheet available until room entered	6 min: assess patient. 3 min: discuss with examiner	Given when 4 min remaining
Safe prescribing	Read task outside room (approx. 2 min)	5 min: write prescription. 4 min: discuss with examiner	Given when 5 min remaining

Most examination centres have lots of helpers at hand to point you in the right direction for your next station. If you become confused or lost as to where you go next simply ask, because time is precious and it will be eating into your 3 minutes of potential preparation time. You will be directed into your next station at the correct time.

The examiners come from a wide variety of clinical backgrounds linked to paediatrics and general practice. Each will have received specific training to assess you in this examination. Often examiners will have been trained to give you no indication of how you are doing. Sometimes their 'blank' expression can be rather off-putting, but persevere and focus on giving a structured, logical answer.

Mark scheme

Each examiner will assess the candidate's performance and allocate a mark of either 'clear pass', 'pass', 'bare fail', 'clear fail' or 'unacceptable' (Table 1.3). Each of these carry a numerical mark. Each station has a specific mark scheme that will be considered in more detail in each respective chapter.

Table 1.3 Description of marks allocated

Mark		Description
Clear pass	12	Competent, satisfies requirements and excels
Pass	10	Good performance, minor errors
Bare fail	8	Inappropriate number of minor or important errors
Clear fail	4	Poor performance
Unacceptable	0	Unprofessional behaviour or very poor performance

There will be 12 objective assessments made of each candidate during the entire eight stations. A total minimum score 120 marks is required to pass the DCH Clinical examination.

Previous paediatric training

It is recommended, but not a prerequisite, that UK candidates sitting the exam have at least 6 months' hospital experience in paediatrics. However, candidates from Hong Kong are required to have 6 months' paediatric experience. Candidates without any paediatric experience are at a disadvantage, but with focused and dedicated preparation it is not insurmountable.

Preparation tips

Given that this is a clinical assessment, you must practise, practise, practise and practise some more! You should aim to have a clear revision schedule at least 6 weeks prior to the examination. This is particularly important because it can be difficult to organize your clinical commitments and those of various paediatric ward rounds or community paediatric clinics. Unless you contact the right people early, you may find that you do not have enough time to gain the required exposure and experience.

You can practise your role-play skills with colleagues, patients, family members, or even alone in front of the mirror. The key is for you to achieve plenty of practise, particularly of your systems examinations, developmental assessment and clinical scenarios. You should seize every opportunity as a learning experience. For example, if a young mother comes in for her repeat prescription of the oral contraceptive pill and has her young child with her, take a moment to assess the child's developmental age and then ask how old the child is. Even if you are waiting at a bus stop or doing your grocery shopping, look out for learning opportunities and assess the developmental ages of the children around you. Practise makes perfect!

For each case, you may wish to practise an opening sentence or two by way of introduction. This may sound odd because you obviously don't know which cases come up, but practising this technique will help you sound more confident on the day, whatever this case may be.

Summary tips

- Start practising early
- Have your revision schedule ready at least 6 weeks before the exam
- Attend as many general and community paediatric clinics as possible
- Practise, practise, practise!

2

COMMUNICATION STATIONS

Communication skills are essential to any doctor–patient interaction. In paediatric cases, communication often takes place with the parents or primary carer, which has inherent pros and cons. On the positive side, this makes it possible to obtain a history and have adult discussions about important issues. On the negative side, however, parents are often very anxious if their child is unwell and this can impact heavily on the consultation. For example, they may forget most of the information you tell them, so it is vital that you summarize, 'safety net' by offering suitable support and follow up, and offer written literature to reinforce your discussion.

This station assesses your ability to communicate effectively, obtain a thorough history and provide accurate information. The examiner will have a brief discussion with you after the case and may ask details about the history or about your subsequent management plan.

Format

There are two separate communication stations, each lasting 6 minutes. You will be given the scenario to read approximately 2 minutes prior to entering the station. The relative lack of reliable child actors means that these stations often involve dealing with a role player, who may be a parent, carer or healthcare professional. You will be asked to conduct your consultation with the role player and/or child. A telephone conversation, such as a call from a concerned parent, doctor or professional may be included. The role player will have brief covering information about the history and specific questions to ask.

You should aim to complete the station within the allocated 6 minutes, however, some of the scenarios might easily form the basis of a 10-minute consultation in general practice. Therefore, candidates are expected to do their best in the given timeframe, because it is possible to pass the station without completing all possible items provided that you communicate appropriately, provide correct information without jargon, suitably close the consultation and arrange appropriate follow up with the role player.

How to approach this station

First and foremost, you should appear calm and welcoming. Greet the role player and/or child appropriately and make them feel at ease. You should introduce yourself clearly and address the role player and/or child as per their name(s) on the brief. Although it can sometimes be tempting, avoid shortening their name or using a 'nickname' to address the child.

You should clearly outline the reason for the consultation and it is helpful to recap the information given on your brief as a starting point. Allow the role player plenty of time to speak and, unless inappropriate, engage the child too. Try not to interrupt when the parent is telling you about the problem; they may well give you more of the answer, plus it is considered rude to interrupt! Always explore the role player's ideas, concerns and expectations. You should discuss pros, cons and alternatives of any course of action, and avoid being judgemental. It is important to remember that, no matter how good your communication skills are, some clinical knowledge is needed to manage these stations. Therefore, when offering advice, it should be accurate and clear. You should avoid jargon and explain terms if necessary.

Always remember to summarize and recognize opportunities to check understanding or offer to answer questions as you go along. This is particularly important, as you may run out of time at the end. When wrapping up the consultation, offer some written material such as a leaflet or website address if appropriate and offer further/continuing support or a follow-up appointment. Where parents are having difficulties with small children, or if you have any concern for the welfare of the child, a follow-up home visit (for example) by the health visitor or other appropriate professional can be arranged.

Top tips

- Build a good rapport
- Display positive and open body language
- Speak clearly and loud enough for the examiner to hear
- Ask concise questions
- Use a mixture of open and closed questions
- Encourage the parent and/or child to speak
- Detect non-verbal and verbal cues
- Avoid jargon
- Summarize the history and discussion

Common themes

The Royal College of Paediatrics and Child Health (RCPCH) highlight six main patterns of communication scenario:

1. **Information giving** (e.g. please explain the diagnosis to the parent)
2. **Consent** (e.g. please obtain consent for a lumbar puncture procedure to be performed)
3. **Critical incident** (e.g. please talk to the parent of a child who has been given a drug he is allergic to)
4. **Ethics** (e.g. please discuss the problem as the child has refused to have any blood tests)
5. **Education** (e.g. please explain the importance of child safety in the home)

6. **Use of common medical devices** (e.g. please explain how to use a steroid nasal spray, a salbutamol inhaler or a peak expiratory flow meter. A mannequin or model may be used in such a station)

From these six patterns, the potential scenarios are endless! However, the basic principles behind each communication station are very similar. Apply the principles outlined earlier and your own clinical experience to each communication station. You will soon find that you are equipped with all the necessary skills to tackle any scenario thrown at you.

Examples of some common topics include: febrile convulsion, nocturnal enuresis, vaccinations, insulin-dependent diabetes, epilepsy counselling, asthma and eczema.

Skills to demonstrate

Use the Anchor statements (pp. 34–35), reproduced with permission from the RCPCH, to understand what the examiners will be looking for. You can use it as a 'mark scheme' to grade your performance when doing the practice cases.

Worked examples and practice cases

The scenarios that follow test clinical knowledge and different aspects of communication and applied knowledge. You should role play scenarios such as these in timed conditions, and generate further role play based on any issues that you may encounter or have difficulty with.

The following cases have been subdivided using the six main patterns of communication scenario as highlighted by the RCPCH.

Information giving

> **Role**: You are a GP
> **Setting**: GP surgery
> **Scenario**: Mrs Jones has come to see you because her daughter Jane, aged 3, was recently admitted to Accident and Emergency (A&E) with a febrile convulsion

As with all such consultations, a recap on what has happened will yield useful material for discussion. You should also ask what advice they were given on admission and discharge.

The main aims of the consultation are to: reassure the parents about the benign nature of the disorder and educate them about prognosis, causes and what to do if it recurs, so that they are not overly anxious about febrile illness in children. The main issues regarding febrile seizures are as follows:

- They are the most common seizure disorder. They are defined as occurring between 6 months and 6 years of age
- Children generally have a normal cognitive and developmental outcome
- They recur in one-third of children and are associated with a low risk of epilepsy (less than 1%)

You should:

- **Assess risk factors for epilepsy**: complex febrile seizure, neurological abnormality and family history of epilepsy
- **Determine whether Jane's seizure was complex**. Complex seizures are defined by at least one of: duration longer than 15 minutes, multiple seizures within 24 hours and focal features

Where a seizure lasts longer than 5 minutes, an ambulance should be called (or a local doctor/paramedic in remote locations). If seizures recur before a child has returned to normal, the child needs to be sent to hospital and rectal diazepam or buccal midazolam may need to be given. Where a child has recurrent febrile convulsions, parents (and possibly nursery staff) can be instructed on the administration of rectal diazepam.

Paracetamol and ibuprofen are often useful in relieving the discomfort of a febrile child, but there is no direct evidence that rigorous reduction of temperature reduces the recurrence of seizures. Tepid sponging is another method of controlling temperature that gives parents a greater sense of participation in the care of a febrile child, however the evidence base to support tepid sponging is not strong.

Role: You are a GP

Setting: GP surgery

Scenario: Mr Pope has brought his 2-year-old son, Alexander, to see you. Alexander has had vomiting and diarrhoea for 2 days. At the local Emergency Medical Department they were told 'to visit you the following day'

Establish what Mr Pope was told about Alexander's diarrhoea, what advice he was given and what the symptoms were attributed to. You may wish briefly to recap on the symptoms:

- What is the nature of the stool (bloody? watery?) and how often is Alexander passing a motion?
- Is he passing less urine? When was the last wet nappy? Has he lost any weight?
- How often and for how long has he been vomiting? Is he taking fluids or paracetamol?
- Does he have any history of major health problems or previous hospital admissions?
- Has anyone else at home been sick?
- Has there been any change in his diet?
- Has he recently travelled abroad?

This scenario (if there are no worrying symptoms) is about reassuring the parent, whilst laying an appropriate safety net should things get worse:

- Gastroenteritis is the most common cause of diarrhoea and vomiting. As it is mostly caused by viruses, antibiotics are of no use
- Treatment is supportive, and the symptoms usually resolve within 1 week. Paracetamol is advocated more for symptoms of pain, distress or lethargy rather than for a fever per se

- If the parents are worried, they can always bring him back or call for help if he is poorly out of hours. If he becomes unresponsive, unrousable, has a fit, displays fear of the light, has an abnormal posture or any symptom that makes his parents very worried, they should consider taking him straight to the nearest A&E department
- Oral rehydration solution (Dioralyte) is available over the counter at chemists. Consider discussing signs of dehydration such as passing less urine
- Sometimes children with diarrhoea may develop transient lactose intolerance
- Breast feeds should be continued for babies with vomiting and diarrhoea.

The history and counselling just given is for acute diarrhoea. Chronic diarrhoea in an infant is also a potential scenario that might bring a parent to see a GP. Try to differentiate between the four main causes of chronic diarrhoea: toddler diarrhoea, secondary cow's milk/lactose intolerance, coeliac disease and cystic fibrosis.

> **Role**: You are a GP
> **Setting**: GP surgery
> **Scenario**: Mrs Papas has come to see you because her son Nicholas, aged 6, was recently admitted overnight with an anaphylactoid reaction to peanuts

It may be useful to recap on what has happened:

- What was done in hospital, what medications were prescribed (is he taking Piriton and prednisolone?)
- What follow up has been advised?
- Did Nicholas have a previous history of atopy, such as eczema, asthma or hay fever? (Most fatal reactions to food occur in people with asthma. Asthma should be optimally controlled)

In IgE-mediated food allergy (such as in this case) common triggers include eggs, milk, peanuts and fish (including seafood); less common triggers include fruit, vegetables and tree nuts. Reactions typically occur within minutes of ingesting the food. They are typically local: angioedema (swelling), perioral itching, laryngeal oedema (sore throat and noisy breathing), and systemic: urticarial rash, soreness of eyes and nose, wheeze, diarrhoea and vomiting and, in some cases, anaphylaxis.

Has Nicholas had any previous investigations for food allergy? Ask about food-specific skin prick tests. For those in whom true food allergy is suspected, or for whom the diagnosis cannot be safely excluded, serum-specific IgE tests to the foods implicated can be performed. Indiscriminate testing is not recommended as tests have low specificity.

Attempt to distinguish true allergy from food intolerance. In food intolerance, symptoms are typically non-specific, making it difficult to establish a temporal relationship between food and symptoms, and at times the foods may be well tolerated. IgE-mediated food allergy will require complete avoidance of the provoking foods. Help from a paediatric dietician with detailed written strategies on food avoidance is useful. Advise scrutiny of the ingredients on packaged cakes and ready meals.

Nicholas needs to be referred to an allergy specialist and ought to have the serum-specific IgE tests while waiting to be assessed (the paediatricians may already have arranged this). Advise the patient/parents that the food triggers should be avoided completely. For patients who have had life-threatening symptoms, prescribe a self-administered epinephrine auto-injector (EpiPen). Patients/parents will need a detailed written plan advising them when and how to use this. The school (alert the school nurse) may also need advice and training. Many hospital resuscitation officers offer training sessions for parents following an anaphylactic reaction in their child.

Offer written information on allergy and anaphylaxis; websites such as www. anaphylaxis.org may offer further information. A Medicalert bracelet may also be useful (www.medicalert.org.uk).

> **Role**: You are a GP
> **Setting**: GP surgery
> **Scenario**: Mrs Thomas would like some advice about her 3-year-old, John. While bathing him, she has noticed that his foreskin is not retractile. He seems obsessed with his penis and his childminder has noticed him playing with himself. Should he have a circumcision operation?

The foreskin is normally not retractile for the first year and is non-retractile for 60% of 6-year-olds because of physiological adhesions, which resolve on their own. Retraction of the foreskin may be attempted in 6-year-old boys for hygiene purposes, but not to tear adhesions, which can cause scarring. Circumcision is rarely medically indicated, and there is intense debate over whether cultural circumcision is an abuse of children's rights.

You can offer to see John. In all likelihood his obsession with his own genitals is normal and will pass – if it does not, further discussion is needed. Circumcision is reserved for especially troublesome symptoms:

- Recurrent balanitis (>3 attacks; the usual treatment is with antibiotic ointment only)
- Phimosis (uncommon). Only consider circumcision if there is difficulty in voiding (ballooning is not an indication). Almost all physiological tightness of the foreskin resolves on its own
- Paraphimosis should be reduced as soon as possible (reduce swelling of the glans with ice) and, if this is not possible, the child should be referred as an emergency
- Excessive amounts of (redundant) foreskin causing irritation and discomfort

Doctors who perform circumcisions should be able to take informed consent from, ideally, both parents and to manage postoperative pain (the main complication). Older children may demonstrate 'Gillick competence' (i.e. be able to understand, consider and retain relevant information), may also be able to give consent and should be consulted. Circumcision of children who are still in nappies can result in ulceration of the urethral meatus and subsequent urethral strictures. In all likelihood, reassurance and some printed information will suffice unless there is a specific indication.

You may also wish to consider how you might discuss circumcision for a child with parents who would like to arrange this for cultural or religious reasons.

> **Role**: You are a GP
> **Setting**: GP surgery
> **Scenario**: Mrs Freeley has come to discuss her son,
> Peter, aged 8. He wets the bed most nights. He has been
> dry during the day since he was 4. The only treatment that
> he has ever had was desmopressin for a sleepover at a
> friend's house, when he was aged 7. In 6 months the family
> are going on a long holiday to Canada

Bed wetting (nocturnal enuresis) is a common issue for young children: 10% of 5-year-olds and 5% of 10-year-olds wet the bed. Enquire into the family circumstances; this may illuminate the cause or affect management. History is crucial: Has the child ever been dry? If the answer is yes, then a cause needs to be found: this might be a urine infection or a first presentation of diabetes mellitus. It could also be a manifestation of bullying or abuse. Is the child dry at night or dry during the day? Specific treatment is often unnecessary for those under the age of 7 years who have never been dry. About 1% of children with wetting have an organic problem. Daytime urinary symptoms in a bed-wetting child suggest an underlying bladder dysfunction. Diabetes, urinary tract infection (UTI), constipation and structural anomalies should be excluded.

It should be emphasized that once a physical problem is ruled out, Peter has a very good chance of achieving dry nights in the long term. However, lasting benefit will require motivation by both Peter and his family. A further appointment for the parents and their son is mandatory, as well as referral if feasible to the local enuresis clinic. Printed information helps. The ERIC website is a valuable resource for parents worried about their child's continence: http://www.eric.org.uk.

Enuresis alarms are effective and safe, but do require several months of continual use and may disrupt family sleep. Desmopressin improves bedwetting in the short term, but relapse occurs on stopping without other management. Oral desmopressin may be an option for travel, short holidays and sleepovers. As of April 2007, this indication for desmopressin as a nasal spray is no longer recommended, but tablets are still in use. Imipramine (an antidepressant) is no longer recommended because of a high risk of serious adverse effects in overdose.

> **Role**: You are a GP
> **Setting**: GP surgery
> **Scenario**: Mrs Shzerpanik would like to obtain some
> 'strong steroid cream' for her daughter Laura, aged 2.
> Laura has had some patches of rough dry skin behind
> her knees and in front of her elbows. She also wants to
> know about medicated bubble baths

A brief recap and history may be useful, as will a brief explanation of the implicit problem. Is there a family history of asthma, eczema or hay fever? Did Laura have eczema on her face or nappy rash as a baby? What has the family tried so far? Have there been any changes at home or any new pets?

Eczema is a longstanding inflammation of the skin, often associated with a family history. It causes intense itching, is made worse by scratching and mainly affects the face, and elbow and knee flexures in toddlers. About 12–15% of children are affected by allergic eczema (avoid the use of 'atopy' in consultations as you will have to waste time explaining it.) The good news is that three-quarters of children grow out of it by the age of 15 years. Scratching and rubbing actually cause most of the clinical signs. Sleep may be affected and children with eczema are sometimes hyperactive. Untreated it can cause skin damage, which sometimes results in teasing and bullying at school, and in toddlers it may even affect growth (if severe). Eczema is prone to infection with bacteria and with certain viruses – if parents suspect this they should bring their child to the GP to be checked. Skin-prick tests or blood tests for specific allergens may be useful only if specific triggers for allergy are suspected. If the rash ever looks red or sore and infected, then swabs may be useful to check for infection to guide the use of antibiotics.

General measures

- By now you will have explained what eczema is and offered a printed leaflet from Patient UK, the British Association of Dermatologists or the National Eczema Society (www.eczema.org). The good prognosis will have been mentioned
- Children should wear loose cotton clothing and avoid wool (which irritates affected skin) and excessive heat
- Nails should be kept short
- Cats and dogs tend to make eczema worse; ideally keep the child away from them
- House dust mite is a factor but is difficult completely to remove from the home
- Avoid soaps and bubble baths (these can be drying and irritants, especially if scented)
- First-line treatment is with emollients. Regular use of aqueous cream and emulsifying ointments (and as soap substitutes) may help. Mrs Shzerpanik could also use a bath oil emollient
- An antihistamine may help, especially with itching at night
- Second-line treatment is with topical steroids – doctors should prescribe the least potent effective ointment (e.g. 1% hydrocortisone BD). Stronger doses may be needed in flare-ups
- Treat secondary infection promptly
- Consider dermatology referral once the above have been tried without success

Should Laura avoid wheat?

Some children with atopic eczema and a history that is suggestive of food allergy (such as mouth rashes, stomach aches, relationship between a foodstuff and symptoms) should avoid the offending food. Dietary exclusion may also be tried when eczema is resistant to other therapies, but the child should have been referred by this point. A paediatric dietician should be involved to make sure the offending food is excluded but dietary deficiencies are avoided in a growing child.

Role: You are a GP

Setting: GP surgery

Scenario: You are asked to see Jenny Smith, a 16-year-old schoolgirl with acne on her forehead, chin and back. Washing with coal tar soap 'smells awful and hasn't helped at all'. Advise her

---

Introduce yourself and briefly recap, checking where she has spots (assessing severity) and exploring her ideas, concerns and expectations. Emphasize that this condition is extremely common in teenagers.

Are there any social pressures such as bullying or romantic frustration? Has she complied with treatment so far? Explore her ideas on personal hygiene. There are many (commercially available) antiseptic soaps that are more pleasant than coal tar. She should try and avoid touching, scratching or 'popping' her spots if she wants to avoid scarring.

You would like to promote a healthy lifestyle and hygiene, however, it may be useful to dispel the myths that acne severity is related to bad diet or poor hygiene. There is no evidence to support this.

There are several approaches to treatment. Many GPs adopt a stepwise approach to treatment, with 2–3 months at each 'step'. The first step is soap and over-the-counter gels and lotions. The second step is topical treatments, such as benzoyl peroxide, which also comes in combination with topical erythromycin or clindamycin. Emphasize that oral antibiotics may appear to have 'cured her best friend overnight', but topical treatments should be tried first unless acne is very severe. Some GPs offer a topical retinoid, such as differin, further down the line, but this can have adverse effects such as photosensitivity and drying of the skin.

As a next step she could be treated with an antibiotic (erythromycin or tetracycline). It is worth mentioning that these also take time to work and can have side effects, such as (for tetracyclines) stomach upset, allergies and sensitivity to sunlight. If, however, an antibiotic is not effective within 3 months, she could (girls only) be prescribed Dianette in addition. You need to explain that Dianette is a contraceptive and may cause headache or breast tenderness. There is an increased risk of deep venous thrombosis. If acne disappears with antibiotics and/or Dianette, the antibiotics are weaned off, then the Dianette should be stopped and the gel may be left as a prophylactic.

If all fails and she has bad acne, she may be asked if she would like to be referred to a 'skin specialist' to be assessed in clinic for other treatments that may have more side effects and are not started by GPs (e.g. roaccutane). Printed information and advice for acne may be helpful. Agree on a plan and a sensible follow-up period.

> **Role**: You are a GP
>
> **Setting**: GP surgery
>
> **Scenario**: Mrs Sanders has come to discuss her 14-year-old daughter, Hermione. Hermione has, for over a year, been missing school on average once a week with terrible stomach aches. She has had numerous ultrasounds, blood tests and at one point a CT looking for appendicitis (these were all normal)

It is hard to distinguish functional abdominal pain from organic abdominal pain. Only the presence of alarm symptoms or signs increases the probability of an organic disorder and justifies further diagnostic testing:

- Involuntary weight loss
- Deceleration of linear growth
- Gastrointestinal blood loss
- Significant vomiting
- Chronic severe diarrhoea
- Unexplained fever
- Persistent right upper or right lower quadrant pain
- Family history of inflammatory bowel disease.

Diagnostic triage to discriminate functional abdominal pain from organic disorders in young people aged 4–18 years with chronic abdominal pain can be carried out by a GP by means of assessment of alarm symptoms or signs and physical examination. Additional diagnostic evaluation is not required in children without alarm symptoms. Testing may be carried out to reassure children and their parents.

Treatment will have to take place over several consultations. If the condition suddenly deteriorates, she may need to be assessed in A&E. Treatment should:

- Deal with psychological factors (consider referral to a paediatric clinical psychologist)
- Educate the family (an important part of treatment)
- Focus on return to normal functioning rather than on the complete disappearance of pain
- Prescribe drugs judiciously as part of a multifaceted, individualized approach, to relieve symptoms and disability

More information can be obtained from the International Foundation for Functional Gastro-intestinal Disorders (www.aboutkidsgi.org/)

> **Role**: You are a GP
>
> **Setting**: GP surgery
>
> **Scenario**: Mrs Smith has come to discuss her son William, aged 6. He has always been an active boy and this sometimes caused difficulties at nursery. Now a primary school teacher has suggested that he might have attention-deficit hyperactivity disorder (ADHD). Advise her

GPs are often the first to be approached first by a concerned parent anxious to know if a poorly performing or badly behaved child has a developmental problem or needs extra help.

There is no biological marker (blood test or scan) that currently identifies children with ADHD. A GP is not in a position to diagnose ADHD – many of the behaviours associated with ADHD are seen in normal children! Screen for:

- **Inattention:** poor attention to detail and organization of tasks, appears not to listen, easily distracted, forgetful, lack of concentration on a given task
- **Impulsiveness:** Shouts out answers to questions, difficulty in taking turns or queuing, talks over others, lack of social awareness
- **Hyperactivity:** fidgets, does not stay in seat, inappropriate running or climbing

Diagnosis requires several such behaviours to be present in more than one setting (e.g. home and school) for >6 months. You should also consider a formal school report. Prior to further referrals it is accepted practice to request a hearing test. Sensitive inquiry into family and domestic circumstances may yield reasons for odd behaviour and this could be followed up in further consultations. You should also consider sensitive screening questions for autism, Asperger syndrome and the autistic spectrum. As with other childhood educational and development problems, if there are any clinical grounds or parental anxiety, then a referral may be made to child psychiatry or community paediatrics (this depends on local arrangements).

Role: You are a GP

Setting: GP surgery

Scenario: Mrs Brown has come for the result of a CT scan, which was organized in a hurry when her daughter, Sophie, aged 3, was found to be unsteady (ataxic) and poorly coordinated at a visit for another problem. The CT shows 'a large posterior fossa lesion highly suggestive of an astrocytoma'

There is no doubt that 5 minutes is not an appropriate length of time in which adequately to break this news. In reality the scan would have probably accompanied an urgent referral. Also, an in-depth knowledge of childhood cancers is not mandatory. The candidate would be expected to understand that extreme bad news is being given to a parent, and to break the bad news appropriately, establishing the parent's ideas, concerns and expectations at the outset. The candidate would also be expected to have a basic idea of what the next steps would involve.

Breaking bad news effectively calls for you to:

- Ask the receptionist to hold your calls/indicate that this is so
- Introduce yourself to the parent
- Find out if anyone else is with her or if she would like them present
- Recap on what has happened – this is a good way to establish ideas, concerns and expectations
- Offer the warning shot: 'The scan result is back, and I'm afraid it is not good news'

- Break the bad news. Avoid using confusing or misleading words like 'lesion' or 'growth', especially if the likelihood is 'cancer' (this is unambiguous)
- Acknowledge that you have given her difficult news, and ask if she understands what you have said and if she has any questions?
- You may have time to go on to 'what happens next', which is itself a likely question from the parent

Whilst a detailed knowledge of paediatric tumours is not essential, that of a broad approach to intracranial problems in children certainly is. Sophie can (if not already) be referred urgently to a 'brain specialist' and a 'children's cancer specialist', who will advise on the next steps. Tests that may need to be done include an electroencephalogram (EEG), skull X-ray, computed tomography (CT) and/or magnetic resonance imaging (MRI) scans, and blood tests. Treatment depends on these further tests and specialist advice, and may involve surgery or medication. Most importantly, you and the practice will continue to offer Sophie and her family support. A follow-up appointment should take place in the next few days. Printed advice and contact details for a relevant self-help group may be valuable also.

Role: You are a GP

Setting: GP surgery

Scenario: Miss Clare Wilcock has brought her 1-month-old girl, Ruby, to see you. She apparently has been vomiting after every feed for the last 2 weeks

---

The standard advice about recapping and eliciting the mother's ideas, concerns and expectations applies here. You should express a wish to examine the baby.

Gastro-oesophageal reflux disease (GORD) is the commonest cause of vomiting in infancy. The vomiting may commence soon after birth but is more frequently delayed for a few weeks. The clinical features are:

- Vomiting usually occurs after a feed, when a small amount of food is regurgitated. From then until the next feed regurgitation may continue
- At times the vomiting may be forceful and may even be 'projectile'
- Vomit is never bile-stained but may contain frank or altered blood or mucus. Bile-stained vomit implies a surgical cause – particularly volvulus – until proven otherwise
- Most infants with this condition thrive normally and are not distressed by it, although it can cause growth restriction
- There may be aspiration of milk – this presents with cough and wheezing

Diagnosis is usually based on the clinical presentation. Differentials include: congenital hiatus hernia, gastroenteritis, pyloric stenosis and UTI.

Management involves:

1. Reassure and advise adequate winding and smaller, more frequent feeds. Raising the head of the crib has been shown to be of uncertain benefit. This occurrence usually resolves spontaneously when the baby reaches the age of 12–18 months. It is recommended that babies who posset are laid on their backs (see cot death advice) to sleep

2. Advise thickened feeds, e.g. Carobel, SMA Staydown
3. Ranitidine and Gaviscon are licensed in infancy, omeprazole and domperidone may be used but are unlicensed
4. Metoclopramide may help symptoms, but must be balanced against possible side effects such as dystonia

GORD complicated by failure to thrive should receive shared care between primary and secondary care. Surgery may be indicated if there is failure to thrive, oesophageal ulceration and recurrent or persistent aspiration.

Common causes of persistent vomiting in all age groups include:

- Posseting
- Overfeeding (a HV's input may help)
- Oesophageal reflux
- Pyloric stenosis (true projectile vomit in 2–6-week-olds who remain hungry)
- Chronic occult infection (e.g. urinary tract infection)
- Intermittent obstruction (e.g. malrotation or volvulus)
- Raised intracranial pressure (sudden/no nausea)
- Migraine (often with family history/headache/aura, etc.)
- Peptic ulcer (with upper abdominal pain)

> **Role**: You are a GP
> **Setting**: GP surgery
> **Scenario**: You have just performed a 6-week-check on Mrs Langdon's firstborn, James. You note that he has prominent epicanthal folds, low-set ears and a single palmar crease. On listening to his heart, you can hear a pansystolic murmur. Discuss your findings with the mother

The implication is the clinical suspicion that James has Down syndrome, and it would be unfair to expect a candidate to cover every aspect of this diagnosis and its implications in 5 minutes. As ever, there are marks for ascertaining the parent's ideas, concerns and expectations. *Beware:* Feelings of intense disappointment, guilt, anger and denial may be elicited by such a diagnosis.

Do not forget to congratulate Mrs Langdon on her new baby. Look at the baby and refer to James by name. Despite the majority of findings were entirely normal, a couple of things in the examination are of concern to you (the warning of possible bad news). 'These findings are sometimes associated with Down syndrome. Do you have any experience of this condition?', is one way of breaking the news. Try and avoid bombarding the parent with information, and let them ask questions.

The diagnosis is not based purely on characteristic appearance. Clinical suspicion must be confirmed by a senior paediatrician. The blood test (for chromosome analysis) for the parents and the baby takes about a week to come back. It is in James's and his family's interests for his result to be known: for reassurance or for knowledge about the possible implications for James's health and wellbeing, and whether there is an increased risk of any future siblings being affected. There is also assistance and support available in the event of a positive diagnosis: from the practice, self-help groups and, if necessary, social support and benefits.

What happens next? Referral to an appropriate paediatrician, genetic counselling and chromosomal analysis blood tests should be the next steps. Remember that at this stage there is no firm diagnosis.

Implications of a diagnosis of Down syndrome include:

- **Immediate/short term**: possible heart defects, duodenal atresia, developmental delay, possible low IQ (this varies – average 50), hearing and eyesight problems
- **Later medical complications**: increased risk of chest infections, hypothyroidism, early-onset Alzheimer disease, atlantoaxial instability and leukaemia
- **However**: life expectancy and quality of life are constantly improving – and issues in the long term may be finding suitable employment and accommodation in adulthood.

Consent

> **Role**: You are a GP
> **Setting**: GP surgery
> **Scenario**: Mrs Killpatrick has booked an emergency appointment with you. While cleaning Kirsten's, her 15-year-old daughter's, room she has found a used packet of Microgynon 30 ED. She is distressed and angry. Your notes show that a partner in the surgery felt that Kirsten was competent to make the decision, and Kirsten asked that her parents were not informed

Contraception, Young People and Confidentiality: The GMC guidance 0–18, which came into force on 13 October 2007, is *mandatory reading*. The following advice is distilled from the GMC guidance.

In this case you are *not allowed* to discuss any part of Kirsten's health record without her explicit consent. The exception would be if you suspected abusive or seriously harmful sexual activity (presumed so in any child under the age of 13). However, you can discuss Mrs Killpatrick's concerns and worries, talk to Kirsten's usual doctor and find out from Mrs Killpatrick whether she suspects an abusive sexual relationship (essentially the discussion you might have in the absence of the notes and any foreknowledge of the absent patient). You might ask: 'Has Kirsten's behaviour changed recently? Is she doing OK at school? Has she got a new group of friends or a boyfriend? Have you had any recent discussions with her about what's going on in her life?'

Stating that you did not prescribe her the pill may itself be considered a breach of confidentiality. Information should be shared about sexual activity if:

- A young person is too immature to understand or consent
- There are big differences in age, maturity or power between sexual partners
- A young person's sexual partner has a position of trust

- There is force or the threat of force, emotional or psychological pressure, bribery or payment, to engage in sex or to keep it secret
- Drugs or alcohol are used to influence a young person to have sex, when otherwise they would not
- Sex involves a person known to the police or child protection agencies as a child abuser

Contraception, abortion and advice and treatment for sexually transmitted infections may be given without parental knowledge to children under the age of 16 years provided that:

- They understand the advice and its implications
- You cannot persuade them to tell or allow you to tell the parents
- There is likelihood of sex without treatment
- Physical or mental health will suffer without advice or treatment
- It is in 'best interests' to receive advice or treatment without parental knowledge

The above points are often referred to as the Fraser Guidelines, and have been incorporated into the Sexual Offences Act 2003. This must not be confused with 'Gillick competence', which refers to the legal principle that children may consent to any treatment provided that they are able to understand, think about, and retain information and use it to come to a decision in a mature manner.

The GMC advice is that consultations should be kept confidential even if treatment or advice has not been provided. At age 16 it is legally presumed that young people have the ability to make decisions about the treatment and advice they receive.

> **Role**: You are a GP
> **Setting**: GP surgery
> **Scenario**: You have been asked to see 12-year-old Anna and her mother by the practice nurse. Anna is thin and has had several chest and throat infections in the last year, each time requiring antibiotics. Your colleague, who saw her at the last appointment, suggested getting blood for a full blood count, fasting blood sugar and an erythrocyte sedimentation rate. Anna is scared of needles, and has refused to have the blood test, even with a topical anaesthetic

Issues to consider include:

- How to gain Anna's informed consent (vital clarification on consent issues can be obtained from the General Medical Council's '0–18' guidance)
- Establishing a rapport and the reasons why Anna is afraid
- Explaining to parent and child why the blood test will help
- Enlisting the mother's help to persuade Anna
- Asking Anna's mother if she is happy to hold her daughter's arm steady, or if she would like the practice nurse to
- Explain to Anna how the analgesic cream will help

Critical incident

> **Role**: You are a GP
> **Setting**: GP surgery
> **Scenario**: Mrs Verity Cross is on the telephone angrily demanding to speak to a doctor. She brought her 12-month-old Joey in with a cold yesterday. One of your colleagues advised paracetamol on a 'dose by weight' basis. Instead of '20 mg/kg TDS' he advised '200 mg/kg TDS'. The mistake was spotted by a helpful pharmacist, who advised her to get back in touch with the surgery

Issues to consider include:

- How is Joey now? Offer to review him
- A sincere apology on behalf of the practice, however you cannot comment on the circumstances as you were not there
- Dealing with an angry parent; avoid confrontation
- Offering an appointment with the doctor concerned
- Offering to talk to the practice team about preventing a mistake like this in future
- Offering to put Mrs Cross in contact with the practice manager if she would like to make a formal complaint.

> **Role**: You are a GP
> **Setting**: GP surgery
> **Scenario**: Mr White has come to see you following the birth of his daughter, Savannah, at 33 weeks' gestation. She needed some oxygen at birth and spent a week having tube feeding in the Special Care Unit. Mr White would like to know what problems might lie in the future for her as a result

Prematurity advice

There may be a large number of marks available for finding out Mr White's ideas, concerns and expectations, e.g.:

- She is so small and fragile; how should I hold her?
- Will she grow and be normal?
- Should we let the family visit?
- What should we do if she won't feed?
- How will I/we/her mother cope?
- Is she at risk of cot death?
- What should we do if we are worried about her?

Some of the issues you may wish to raise and explore may tally with the parental anxieties:

- **Feeding difficulties**: The suckling reflex develops between 32 and 36 weeks' gestation. Some babies will struggle initially with feeding, and may need smaller, more regular feeds or support with nasogastric feeding. As they are small they dehydrate easily, fluid balance needs to be maintained
- Premature babies frequently have **gastro-oesophageal reflux** and sometimes an immature gag reflex (this carries a risk of aspiration). Some will need antireflux medication and follow up with a speech and language therapist
- Small and premature babies are at increased risk of **low blood sugar** in the first few days, especially if they have feeding problems. Parents should seek advice if their child is excessively jittery
- Premature birth can be a difficult time for parents, and admission to hospital may interfere with the normal **bonding** between them and their new baby. Parents have difficulty dividing attention between the new baby and any older children. A sensitive question about how things are at home may yield some discussion
- Some premature babies are distressed at birth. Others are more prone to chest infections, bronchiolitis and other chest problems in infancy. Premature babies are also prone to apnoea attacks. Parents should be encouraged to get their child seen if they are worried about their child's breathing
- **Thermoregulation** (hypothermia) – premature babies have an immature temperature control system; it is very important that the baby is kept warm. Kangaroo care, skin-to-skin contact with the mother or father, is claimed to be effective in maintaining temperature and to help with parent–child bonding.
- **Jaundice** of prematurity: 80% of premature babies.
- Premature babies are more at risk of **infection** – maternal antibodies are reduced in the womb and also if they are not breast fed. This includes chest infections, meningitis and necrotizing enterocolitis (there is an increased risk in bottle-fed babies. Necrotizing enterocolitis is also seen in roughly 10% of babies weighing less than 1500 g). Breast feeding should be encouraged in preference to bottle feeding in the absence of contraindications. Find out if the baby's mother was told to avoid breast feeding for any reason
- She may need to be followed up regularly by the ophthalmologist during the first year. This is because sometimes the oxygen needed at birth can affect the blood vessels in the back of the eyes (**retinopathy of prematurity**). When this is severe, early laser surgery may prevent blindness
- Some premature babies are anaemic because their bone marrow is immature or because of the large number of blood tests that they have had in the Special Care Unit (SCU). For this reason they are often given an **iron supplement** to take after leaving the SCU. Late anaemia may also occur
- **Patent ductus arteriosus**: in some premature and full-term babies the ductus does not close. If the baby is breathless, sweaty, pale or blue when feeding, then an urgent opinion should be sought. This is usually picked up on the baby check as a heart murmur at birth or 6 weeks
- There is a slightly increased risk of cot death in premature babies (see advice later)

Conditions that are more common in very premature babies include:

- Intracranial haemorrhage (in the immature brain, the blood vessels are more fragile)
- Very low blood sugar
- Respiratory distress syndrome
- Chronic lung disease (where a child has been ventilated)
- Apnoeas
- Long-term neurodevelopmental problems (follow up needed)
- Deafness (especially if aminoglycoside antibiotics are needed)

Although parents are usually keen to find out as much as possible, the amount of information may be overwhelming.

Sources of support

Premature babies should be reviewed by a paediatrician in clinic and may, depending on their gestation and condition at birth, have a follow-up appointment for a hearing test and a review by an ophthalmologist. Sources of support are the midwife, HV and GP. For those who have been admitted to a special care baby unit or neonatal intensive care unit there should be a telephone number on the discharge letter that parents can ring for advice. There may be a premature baby group for informal support and advice and there are some very good websites such as www.bliss.org.uk.

Disabilities such as cerebral palsy, hearing loss, visual impairment and educational and developmental problems are associated with extreme prematurity. For most preterm infants of >32 weeks' gestation, survival and longer term neurodevelopment are similar to those of infants born at term. Overall, outcomes are also good for infants born after shorter gestations. Most infants survive without substantial neurodevelopmental problems and most go on to attend mainstream schools, ultimately living independent lives.

Ethics

> **Role**: You are a GP
> **Setting**: GP surgery
> **Scenario**: Mrs Smith is worried about her 15-year-old daughter, Sarah. Sarah has been doing less well at school, and yesterday Mrs Smith found some cannabis hidden in her daughter's room. Mrs Smith confesses to having 'smoked dope' in the 70s, but is really worried that Sarah will want to try more dangerous drugs. Sarah does not know her mother is seeing you

Remember: you cannot divulge information about a third party, although you may have to take action if there is a duty of care to someone who lacks capacity. You are unable to discuss Sarah's health record in the absence of explicit consent from Sarah and unless there is compelling reason. You may begin by asking Mrs Smith what her concerns are and finding out more. She may just want to air her worries and you can provide her with some facts and sources of support and advice. A useful website is www.talktofrank.com. The 'Talk to Frank' helpline number is 0800 776600 (UK only).

You may want to ask: 'How is Sarah behaving?' 'What effect is this having at home, with friends or at school?' 'Are there any family, interpersonal or emotional problems?' 'Is there a previous or family history of mental health problems, or is she merely a typical "troubled teenager"'? 'What does she do with her friends, and who does she confide in?'

You may suggest that it is appropriate to invite Sarah for an appointment. Any suggestion that she is not competent or mentally ill should prompt a desire to seek senior advice (and advice from a medical defence provider). Warn Mrs Smith that you may need to talk to Sarah alone if they come together.

Cannabis use is common amongst teenagers in the UK: 10% of under 16s reported using it in 2006. Its possession is still a criminal offence, which may result in confiscation and prosecution. Heavy cannabis use does increase the risk of schizophrenia and depression in susceptible individuals, especially if there is a family history of mental illness. Also, today's cannabis is much stronger than that available in the 1960s and 1970s. Smoking cannabis adds smoking-related risks.

Acknowledge Mrs Smith's concerns – many do believe that cannabis use leads to abuse of other substances and other problems. This is partly because drug use is more common in 11–16-year-olds with ADHD, truancy, depression and other psycho–social disorders. It is also because the drug affects education, work and driving skills, and may lead to less awareness of personal safety, such as vigilance about sexual intercourse or trying other drugs. It can affect the developing brain. Side effects do include paranoia, confusion and anxiety. Explore Mrs Smith's ideas, concerns and expectations in this consultation. Let her know that you are willing to explore local sources of support if necessary, and that you are willing to broach the topic with Sarah at her next consultation.

Education

Health promotion/education and child health advice form an important part of community paediatrics. GPs should be able to offer advice and educate about key topics.

> **Role**: You are a GP
> **Setting**: GP surgery
> **Scenario**: Mrs Smith has just been seen in A&E with 2-year-old Britanny, who has accidentally swallowed some cleaning products. She was in A&E 2 months ago after her 1-year-old burned herself with a cup of tea. Please talk to her about accident prevention

Introduce yourself and put the parent at ease. Acknowledge how difficult it can be looking after toddlers. Does she have any help? Do not blame her; a non-judgemental attitude helps.

Offer to give her some advice to make her home safer. At the age of 2 most children are walking and curious about their environment. This is a potentially accident-prone time! Most accidents (in adults and children) occur in the living room, followed by the kitchen. You should try to find out:

- Is the child adequately supervised, especially when eating or in an area where they can roam and are free to fall or encounter a hazard?
- Are medicines kept locked away and out of reach?
- Are locks fitted on cupboards where knives, medications and cleaning products are stored? Are stair gates and plug sockets covered?
- Are small objects that could be swallowed or aspirated out of reach?
- Are electrical flexes out of reach of curious little hands?
- Are hot pans/stoves, kettles/irons and their cables, and hot drinks out of reach?
- Water safety – care with baths: is water temperature tested, taking care to not leaving the child unattended
- Not smoking (especially indoors) and taking safety measures in the bedroom, i.e. with the 'back to sleep' campaign for babies
- Road safety, car seats, seatbelts.

Offer contact with the HV to visit and check her home/offer advice. Ongoing support may be provided by the GP or HV, and childcare assistance possibilities explored. Useful books, e.g. *Birth to Five*, can be offered. Ask if there are any questions and attempt to answer these. Offer a follow-up visit.

> **Role**: You are a GP
> **Setting**: GP surgery
> **Scenario**: You have been asked to talk to Mr Smith about the measles/mumps/rubella (MMR) vaccination for his boy Johnny, aged 18 months. Though his wife is keen to proceed, Mr Smith has an autistic son, aged 10, by a previous marriage

Warning: Do not become too distracted by issues of parental responsibility while this discussion is taking place. Though the father has parental responsibility, this should be a shared decision. He probably just wants to discuss his concerns. If a parent or third party were actively seeking a treatment for a child and the other parent were known to be objecting to it, this would prompt discussion of parental responsibility and the best interests of the child.

General advice

Ultimately a parent may choose to disagree with you. If so, offer information and the opportunity to return for further discussion.

Introduce yourself and put him at ease, by saying 'What can I do for you today?'

Listen to and acknowledge his ideas and concerns. You may want to ask: 'What in particular concerns you about the MMR vaccine? What have you read? Do you have personal experience of children with autism?'

Do not be judgemental or coercive. You may find it useful to say: 'It is your decision to do what you feel is best for your child.'

Points to address

Scientific evidence linking the MMR vaccine to autism is lacking. The number of cases of autism has been increasing since 1979. There has been no sudden increase with the introduction of the MMR vaccine in the UK in 1988. Several large European studies have found no association between the MMR vaccine and autism.

Autism is commonly diagnosed after 18 months of age as children start to talk and interact. It has a genetic component and associated neurological abnormalities have been seen to start in the womb. The MMR vaccine is given twice: at 13 months and at preschool entry to 'boost' immunity, so parents may sometimes associate the onset of autism with the MMR. The original paper in *The Lancet* by Wakefield et al. described a case series of only 12 children, failed to take the above points into account and has now been discredited.

Known side effects of MMR

Of those who take the MMR vaccine, 10% develop fever, malaise and a rash 5–21 days after the first vaccination; 3% develop painful joints. Special vaccination precautions are needed in children with severe anaphylactic reactions to egg or chronic severe asthma.

Single vaccines

There is no evidence of any benefit. The USA, Canada and 38 European countries use MMR vaccination. Single vaccines mean three times the distress, three visits, a risk of febrile reactions, a longer time taken to establish immunity – and a longer period where the child is unprotected. The single vaccines are not available on the NHS – parents have to pay.

Dangers of non-vaccination

Measles can cause death, pneumonia, deafness and a slow relentless form of encephalitis (subacute sclerosing panencephalitis). Mumps may result in meningitis, pancreatitis and sterility from orchitis. The babies of pregnant women exposed to rubella may suffer congenital rubella syndrome, which causes deafness, blindness, heart problems and brain damage. Measles is contagious. Every child with measles infects 15 others. If <96% of children are immunized (as is now the case in the UK), then an epidemic may occur.

There is a great deal of information to give so Mr Smith may need to come back after having thought about what he has been told. You can offer an information leaflet/website suggestions such as the government website www.mmrthefacts.nhs.uk, which refers to inflammatory bowel disease and autism. Summarize and ask Mr Smith if he has any questions.

Remember there is not much time – keep your advice simple, explore concerns and offer a follow-up appointment, ideally with both parents present. There is no need to refer to an expert except for special vaccination precautions, or if there are ongoing parental concerns.

> **Role**: You are a GP
> **Setting**: GP surgery
> **Scenario**: Mrs Brown has come to see you about her daughter, Georgina, aged 10. The school nurse has voiced concerns that Georgina is significantly overweight (BMI 35). She is being teased and bullied

Remember:

- Plump children are often seen as 'healthy children'; a parent's desire to feed their child is often perceived as instinctive. You may be faced with denial that there is a problem.
- Obesity is an increasing problem in developed countries.
- Overweight children are more likely to be socially isolated and have psychological problems.
- Being overweight is associated with other lifestyle-related diseases in adulthood, including heart disease, diabetes, asthma and cancers of the breast and bowels, as well as osteoarthritis.
- Overweight children are twice as likely to be overweight adults, and this likelihood is higher if a parent is overweight or there is a relapse following weight loss.

Five minutes is enough time to explore the mother's concerns and expectation, and to provide education on what further appointments will involve. You should arrange to see the mother and daughter together, weigh Georgina and plot her weight and height against an appropriate paediatric centile chart. Because of the changes in childhood adiposity, BMI should be interpreted with caution.

You should ask permission to get information from the school as needed. Georgina is still growing, so she must aim to maintain a steady weight or to reduce the speed at which she puts on weight. There is little evidence that 'weight loss' diets and medication actually work. The earlier the intervention, the higher will be the likelihood of success. Though obesity can have a genetic component, it is far more likely that the problem is one of a mismatch between food intake and physical activity. Eating patterns are often set by the child's family, and any proposed treatment must be acceptable to the family. Parents are usually better agents of change than children, and treating parents and children together is more effective than treating children alone.

The mainstay of management is to aim for a balanced diet rather than a restrictive one, avoiding too many energy-dense foods. An appointment with a dietician may be offered. Many parents find a traffic light system of green (can eat as often as wants), amber (mealtimes) and red (rare treat) helpful. A multifaceted approach to childhood obesity is favoured in the recent National Institute for Clinical Excellence (NICE) guidelines. Physical activity should be encouraged, but bear in mind that overenthusiastic exercise may expose a child's obesity, cause embarrassment and be abandoned. Walking and cycling are a good start. The psycho–social consequences of obesity may be the most important for a child.

> **Role**: You are a GP
> **Setting**: GP surgery
> **Scenario**: Mrs Littlejohn would like to discuss her 4-year-old son, John. He is smaller than other children at nursery and is a picky eater. Mrs Littlejohn is of average height

According to popular general practice magazines, about 40% of parents worry about their child's eating. However, children with 'failure to thrive' have a weight below the third centile for their age and a declining growth velocity and/or a drop across two or more centile lines on a growth chart. John needs to have serial measurements of height and weight to make such a diagnosis. Note: A reduced weight compared with a normal head circumference in a seemingly well child is a sign of reduced food intake. It is worth exploring a typical day's intake and suggesting keeping a food diary for a week. Consider offering a printed leaflet from a website such as Patient UK. You need to arrange follow up and to see and examine John.

Consider

Short parents generally have short children. Children's growth pattern may also follow that of their parents (this is called 'constitutional delay'). Other commoner causes that may be explored are:

- Psycho–social problems (are things happy at home?)
- Lactose or cow's milk protein intolerance (does he refuse or have any problems after any particular type of food?)

A brief history should be taken of whether John has tummy aches, longstanding ('chronic' is a word often misinterpreted as severe) diarrhoea, birth weight (small?) and other problems with feeding or health. Lactose intolerance may follow an acute gastrointestinal infection and may persist for months. Cow's milk protein intolerance is rare after the age of 2 years. Suggesting other types of milk or dietary change should not take place at the first consultation unless there is a clear indication.

Rarer causes to bear in mind are: cystic fibrosis, coeliac disease, intrauterine growth restriction, chronic severe asthma and chronic urinary infections.

Note: Consider how to apply a similar approach to a 12-month-old who is failing to gain weight, or a 1-month-old who is 'failing to gain weight' according to the parents.

> **Role**: You are a GP
> **Setting**: GP surgery
> **Scenario:** Mrs Hardwicke would like something for her 8-year-old boy, Jeremy, to 'help him go'. He's been struggling to go to the toilet once every few days. It is now quite painful, he cries at the thought of going to the toilet and his tummy is starting to get tender and bloated

Ask about: Jeremy's diet and fluid intake, his previous bowel habit, and how the parents and child are coping. Find out if he ever has accidents with his bowels or bladder and say that you would like to see Jeremy to 'feel his tummy'.

Acute constipation is caused by:

- Dehydration – fever, hot environment, not drinking
- Bowel obstruction – is sometimes due to congenital malformations, more likely to present as an acute abdomen
- A change of diet or environment (such as a decrease in dietary fibre and fluids)

Laxatives may be required and Movicol is currently 'in fashion' though lactulose can be used. Chronic constipation can be:

- Functional – as is common with disabled children
- Secondary to withholding, such as with an anal fissure

These do respond to treatment with diet and/or laxatives and bowel training. Be aware that chronic constipation may present with overflow diarrhoea or soiling.

Education for the parent includes guidelines from www.childhoodconstipation. com:

- Do not let your child wait to do a poo
- Give your child enough time so that they do not feel rushed. Set time aside each day for your child to sit on the toilet, ideally after meals
- Make going to the toilet fun, with treats such as a favourite book or blowing bubbles
- If 'it hurts to poo', they can stop and try again later
- Lots of active play will increase bowel activity
- Try to include a variety of high-fibre foods in the family's diet, as well as dried fruit, fruit with skin on and vegetables – especially green beans and lentils (these can be puréed for babies)
- Encourage your child to drink 6–8 glasses of water or fruit juice per day (avoid caffeinated fizzy drinks)

Management

Management includes:

- Examination of the abdomen, looking for anal fissures or neurological causes
- Evacuation: diet, laxatives (lactulose/Movicol), rarely enemas, even more rarely manual disimpaction under anaesthesia
- Maintenance with diet/laxative for 3–6 months, allocating regular times a day when a child sits on the toilet for 10–15 minutes
- Following return to normal: vigilance and early use of treatment at the first sign of hard stool
- If the child is deliberately soiling in inappropriate places (encopresis), then refer to a child psychiatrist

> **Role**: You are a GP
> **Setting**: GP surgery
> **Scenario**: Mrs Evans has come in with her 3-week-old boy, Charles. Though she has breast fed thus far, she is finding it hard to keep up with his demands for feeds and is tired. She also complains that her nipples are getting sore, and that she feels uncomfortable feeding Charles in public

Should a patient breast feed?

It is appropriate to state that to examine the cracked nipple an appointment will need to be made with an appropriate chaperone present. Topical remedies such as nipple shields, Kamillosan or even some breast milk can be tried. If there is redness or swelling, topical or oral antibiotics may be needed but these will not harm the baby (oral penicillins are safe).

Advantages to breast feeding include:

- For the first month at least it confers some protection for baby against infection
- Less chance of allergy problems in baby
- Results in better bonding between mother and child
- Cheaper and possibly more convenient than bottle feeding
- Protects mother against breast and ovarian cancer
- Promotes weight loss
- Initially helps control postpartum bleeding

Working women often have problems breast feeding. Some employers are more supportive than others. It is possible to breast feed at home and express enough milk for the following day, but expressing milk and freezing it when the mother is back at work can be tiring.

> **Role**: You are a GP
> **Setting**: GP surgery
> **Scenario**: The HV has asked you to see Mrs Arden. She and her husband lost their first child to cot death 3 years ago. Mrs Arden is anxious about the health of her new baby, Elizabeth, and has not been sleeping, even when Elizabeth is asleep, for fear that she stops breathing

Cot death advice

Parents who have suffered a sudden and unexpected death of a baby often feel anxious when they have another baby. The Foundation for Sudden Infant Death has set up the Care of the Next Infant (CONI) programme to help parents work

CONI HELPS PARENTS TO WORK THROUGH

through some of their fears. CONI is run in hospitals and community health centres and involves midwives, paediatricians, GPs and HVs. Through CONI, parents can:

- Receive weekly home visits by their HV, so they can talk freely about any worries and seek advice
- Keep a symptom diary to record their baby's health, which they can then discuss with their HV
- Monitor their baby's growth with a weight chart and weighing scales, to detect changes quickly
- Borrow apnoea (breathing) monitors, which pick up movements as the baby breathes and will ring an alarm if movements stop for longer than 20 seconds
- Receive a room thermometer and guidance on bedding and clothing

The accepted advice for reducing the risk of cot death is as follows:

- Avoid smoking in pregnancy (including passive smoking)
- Do not smoke in the same room as the baby
- Do not let the baby get too hot
- Keep the baby's head uncovered
- Place the baby in a lying position with back to cot mattress and feet to the foot of the cot (prevents the baby wriggling under blankets) – as advocated by the 'Back to Sleep' campaign
- Keep the cot in the parents' room for first 6 months
- Do not share the bed with the baby if (either) parent is a smoker, has been drinking alcohol, has taken medication that causes drowsiness, or feels very tired
- It is dangerous to sleep together with the baby, whether in a bed or armchair
- If the baby is unwell, seek professional advice promptly (HV, GP, A&E, etc.)

Use of common medical devices

Role: You are a GP

Setting: GP surgery

Scenario: Mrs Doyle has made an urgent appointment to see you regarding her son Len, aged 7. During a recent wheezy episode following a viral illness, one of the partners at your surgery prescribed a steroid inhaler. She does not know how to use it and is worried that it will make his bones brittle, stunt his growth and make him aggressive

You should be aware of the latest BTS Guidelines for Asthma in children under 5 and children aged 5–12. Len needs an inhaler technique demonstration and his management reviewed. There is no evidence to support preventative low-dose corticosteroid use in viral wheeze. You may need briefly to recap to find out if asthma is suspected. Was the medication prescribed for prophylaxis or for the acute episode only? Look for any suspicion of alternative diagnoses: is there wet cough, stridor, voice change or weight loss? Len may not yet be measuring peak flows, but may be able to start this soon.

Assess control of wheeze by determining the following: 1) Is there wheeze or cough?, 2) Are nights distressed?, 3) Has there been absence from school or interference with play and activities?

Assess the frequency of use of his short-acting bronchodilator (blue inhaler), oral steroids or emergency consultations. Ask about possible triggers. If a pattern suggestive of asthma has emerged, then Len needs regular review to assess inhaler technique and measure his growth. Over time an individual asthma management plan needs to be negotiated, including times when medication should be increased and when Len needs to be seen.

Evaluate Mrs Doyle's ideas, concerns and expectations surrounding asthma. Does she understand the role of the 'reliever' and 'preventer'? It is important for the development of a growing boy to have improved exercise tolerance and lung development, and growth may be assisted by an inhaled bronchodilator and/or steroid. Inhaled steroids are given at a very low dose. They are safe provided that they are used appropriately. Used excessively, inhaled steroids may cause problems such as adrenal suppression, which is why supervision over time by a doctor or practice nurse is important. However, osteoporosis is associated with long-term oral steroid use. You may reassure her about the aggression and stunting of growth.

Note: It is also worth having a working knowledge of the diagnosis and management of allergic rhinoconjunctivitis in children, and the role of steroid and decongestant nasal sprays.

Additional practice cases

- A mother comes to see you concerned about her 10-week-old son. She reports that he 'cries non-stop all day' and she is struggling. He feeds well and has normal soft stool and wet nappies. Please advise.
- You need to administer the 8-week immunizations to a baby girl. She is with her mother. Please obtain consent.
- You just had a discussion with the mother of an 11-month-old baby admitted with a cough. You told her that the chest X-ray had shown an infection and that antibiotics are required. However, this was an error. Her baby's chest X-ray was normal, but you had looked at the wrong patient's chest X-ray report. You now need to update the mother and explain the situation.
- An 8-year-old boy fell off his bike and hit his head; he requires a CT head scan. His father is refusing a CT head scan. Discuss this with the father.
- A mother comes to see you with questions about weaning her 6-month-old daughter. Please advise.
- A 16-year-old boy has worsening control of his asthma. You notice that he has a turbohaler, which was last prescribed a year ago. He also uses a peak flow meter intermittently but has no recent readings. Discuss the situation with him.

Anchor statement: communication stations

Stations 1 and 2: Communication skills		
	Expected standard/ CLEAR PASS	**PASS**
RAPPORT	Full greeting and introduction Clarifies role and agrees aims and objectives Good eye contact and posture Perceived to be actively listening (nod etc.) with verbal and non-verbal cues Appropriate level of confidence, empathetic nature, putting parent/child at ease	Adequately performed but not fully fluent in conducting interview
INFORMATION GATHERING	Asks clear questions Patient and examiner can hear and understand fully Mixture of open and closed style Avoids jargon Allows parent/child sufficient time to speak Picks up verbal and non-verbal cues Verifies and summarises parent/child history	Questions reasonable and cover all essential issues but may omit occasional relevant but less important points Overall approach structured Appropriate style of questioning responsive to parent/child Summarizes history

© Royal College of Paediatrics and Child Health 2012, reproduced with permission.

BARE FAIL	CLEAR FAIL	UNACCEPTABLE
Incomplete or hesitant greeting and introduction Inadequate identification of role, aims and objectives Poor eye contact and posture Not perceived to be actively listening (nod etc.) with verbal and non-verbal cues Does not show appropriate level of confidence, empathetic nature or putting parent/child at ease	Significant components omitted or not achieved	Dismissive of parent/child concerns Fails to put parent or child at ease Lack of civility or politeness Inappropriate manner including flippancy
Misses relevant information which if known would make a difference to the management of the problem Excessive use of closed instead of open questions Uses medical jargon occasionally Misses verbal or non-verbal cues Summary inaccurate/incomplete	Asks closed questions instead of open questions Questions poorly comprehended by parent/child Inappropriate use of medical jargon Inappropriately interrupts parent/child Hasty approach Does not seek views of parent or child Poorly structured interview	Shows no regard for parent or child's feelings Rudeness or arrogance No verification or summarizing

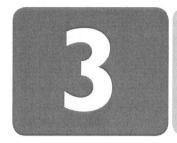

DATA INTERPRETATION

Data interpretation is a crucial part of a doctor's clinical assessment of a patient. It can be particularly important for babies and children, when the history may not be clear.

This station is designed to assess your ability to interpret data in a clinical context, discuss the implications of the data and construct a suitable management plan.

Format

This 6-minute station takes place between you and the examiner. You will not be given any information prior to entering the station. Once the assessment commences, you will be given 2 minutes to interpret the data provided and then have 4 minutes to discuss the implications of the data and your management plan with the examiner.

How to approach this station

Make sure you use the 2 minutes of data interpretation time wisely. Read and understand the data carefully and then deduce your conclusions. You will need to write down your answer to the questions associated with the data. Be logical in your interpretation of the data, and remember that 'common things occur commonly'. If time allows, start thinking about what questions the examiner may ask during the discussion and how you could answer these.

If you cannot understand the data or cannot reach a conclusion about the diagnosis, don't panic! Remain calm and think logically about the scenario and the possible differential diagnoses.

> Top tips
> - Analyse the data carefully
> - Use the clinical context provided within the scenario to help
> - Aim to reach a definitive diagnosis, alternatively list the relevant differential diagnoses
> - Offer the management plan(s) for your diagnosis

Common themes

There are several types of scenario that could arise. Some common themes are:

- Blood tests
- Urinalysis
- Growth charts
- Audiograms
- Peak flow charts
- Diabetic blood glucose diaries

This is not an exhaustive list, but you should be familiar with these at least. Other themes that could come up are interpretation of:

- Family tree diagrams
- Electroencephalograms (EEGs)
- Cerebrospinal fluid (CSF)
- Electrocardiograms (ECGs)
- Blood gases
- Spirometry

Skills to demonstrate

Use the Anchor statements (pp. 50–51), reproduced with permission from the RCPCH, to understand what the examiner will be looking for. You can use it as a 'mark scheme' to grade your performance when doing the practice cases.

Worked examples

The worked examples that follow will help you work through data interpretation scenarios and give you insight into the skills to demonstrate.

1. Peak flow

> ### Candidate information
>
> The task is to interpret the data in the clinical context provided.
> Discuss with the examiner the relevance of the data in terms of diagnosis and management
> This is a 6-minute station. You will have 2 minutes to read the information once you enter the station, and then 4 minutes for discussion with the examiner
> **Role:** You are a GP
> **Setting**: GP surgery
> **Task:** Data interpretation
> **Scenario:** A 7-year-old boy has been suffering with a nocturnal and early morning cough. He also coughs during football training. On examination his chest is clear. His growth charts are normal
> **Investigation:** Peak flow monitoring

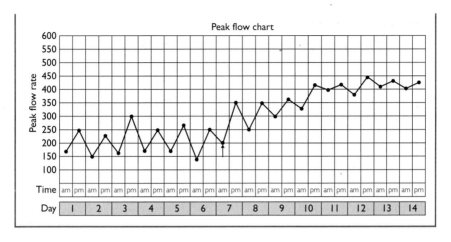

Example questions:

1. What is the likely diagnosis?
2. How does the peak flow chart demonstrate this?
3. What does the arrow at day 7 most likely indicate?
4. How would you manage this child?

Example answers:

1. Asthma
2. Diurnal variation, with lower early morning peak flow readings. This is consistent with his history given in the scenario of nocturnal cough
3. Intervention – treatment with inhaler therapy started. This inhaler is likely a 'preventer' (steroid) inhaler, given the gradual improvement of peak flow readings and reduced diurnal variation during the subsequent week of therapy
4. Continue inhaler therapy. Use a steroid 'preventer' inhaler and salbutamol 'reliever' inhaler. Assess inhaler technique and adequate spacer device. Educate the child and parent(s) about asthma and how to recognize an exacerbation. Reassess the child via an asthma nurse. Refer to the stepwise approach to asthma management in children as per the British Thoracic Society (BTS) guidelines.

Further reading

BTS guidelines: http://www.brit-thoracic.org.uk/guidelines.aspx

2. Urinalysis

> ### Candidate information
>
> **Role:** You are a GP
> **Setting:** GP surgery
> **Task:** Data interpretation
> **Scenario:** A 4-year-old girl is brought by her mother to see you with symptoms of a urinary tract infection (UTI). She has a history of three previous UTIs. She is apyrexial and haemodynamically stable. Urinalysis is as follows
> **Investigation:** Urinalysis
>   **Blood:** Negative
>   **Protein:** Negative
>   **Leucocytes:** Positive
>   **Nitrites:** Positive
>   **Glucose:** Negative
>   **Ketones:** Negative

Example questions:

1. What is the likely diagnosis?
2. How would you manage this patient and why?
3. Would you do any imaging for this patient?

Example answers:

1. Recurrent UTI
2. Start empirical antibiotic therapy for UTI because the urinalysis is positive for both leucocytes and nitrites. Send the urine for MCS (microscopy, culture and sensitivity) to obtain specific sensitivities.
3. Yes, she requires an ultrasound scan within 6 weeks and a dimercaptosuccinic acid (DMSA) within 4–6 months of this infection as per the National Institute for Clinical Excellence (NICE) guidelines for recurrent UTIs in a child over 3 years of age.

Further reading

National Institute for Clinical Excellence. NICE guideline *UTI in Children*: http://www.nice.org.uk/CG54

3. Audiogram

Candidate information

Role: You are a GP
Setting: GP surgery
Task: Data interpretation
Scenario: A mother is concerned about her 3-year-old son's hearing and speech. She had previously seen your colleague, who requested an audiogram. The result of the audiogram is below
Investigation: Audiogram

From: http://www.raisingdeafkids.org/hearingloss/testing/audiogram/ome.php

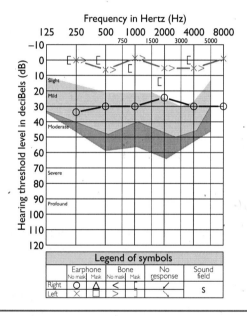

Example questions:

1. What is the probable diagnosis?
2. What are the potential underlying causes?
3. How would you manage this child?

Example answers:

1. Right ear mild to moderate conductive hearing loss
2. Otitis media or glue ear (if glue ear is suspected, consider requesting tympanography)
3. Explain the results to the mother. Treat any underlying active infection or refer to ear, nose and throat (ENT) specialist if indicated for assessment of grommets. Refer to speech and language therapist.

4. CSF

> ### Candidate information
> **Role:** You are a paediatric senior house officer (SHO)
> **Setting:** Paediatric ward
> **Task:** Data interpretation
> **Scenario:** You receive the CSF results for a child who is unwell on the ward
> **Investigation:** CSF
>
> | Test | CSF results | Normal range |
> |------|-------------|--------------|
> | Red cells | 0 | 0 |
> | White cells | Lymphocytes raised | 0–5 WBC |
> | Protein | 30 | 15–60 mg/100 mL |
> | Glucose | 70 | 50–80 mg/100 mL |
> | Appearance | Clear | – |
> | Ziehl–Neelsen stain | Negative | – |

Example questions:

1. What is the diagnosis?
2. Is it a notifiable condition and if so, to whom?
3. The child makes a good recovery; what follow up is required?

Example answers:

1. Viral meningitis
2. Yes, notify the Health Protection Agency (HPA).
3. Though viral meningitis is much less likely than bacterial meningitis to have long-term sequelae, for parental reassurance children are often offered a 6-month follow up and screened for signs of subsequent deafness, seizures or developmental delay.

5. Blood test

> ### Candidate information
> **Role:** You are a GP
> **Setting:** GP surgery
> **Task:** Data interpretation
> **Scenario:** A 4-year-old boy has the following haematology blood results
> **Investigation:** Blood test
>
> | | | |
> |------|------|------|
> | WCC | 5×10^9/L | (4.5–13) |
> | Hb | 9.9 g/dl | (11–17) |
> | MCV | 69 fl | (80–100) |
> | Platelets | 220×10^9/L | (150–450) |

Example questions:

1. What are possible differential diagnoses?
2. What further investigations would you do?
3. How would you manage this patient?

Example answers:

1. Microcytic anaemia due to iron deficiency anaemia, thalassaemia, sideroblastic anaemia
2. Ferritin, total iron binding capacity, blood film. It would be expected to see a low ferritin and high total iron binding capacity in iron deficiency anaemia
3. Depending on the underlying cause. Advise iron supplementation if required. Refer to paediatrician +/– haematologist if underlying haemoglobinopathy is present.

6. Clinical examination

> ### Candidate information
>
> **Role**: You are a GP
> **Setting**: GP surgery
> **Task**: Data interpretation
> **Scenario**: A 3-week-old baby girl is brought to see you with sweating and difficulty feeding. Your examination reveals the following
> **Interpretation**: Clinical examination
>   **Appearance**: no cyanosis
>   **Cardiovascular**: Tachycardia, bounding peripheral pulses, no radio-femoral delay, continuous machinery murmur
>   **Respiratory**: Tachypnoea
>   **Gastrointestinal**: No organomegaly, no ascites

Example questions

1. What is the probable diagnoses?
2. How would you manage this patient?
3. What further investigations would you expect them to do?
4. What are the management options for this condition?

Example answers:

1. Patent ductus arteriosus
2. Urgent referral to Paediatric Accident and Emergency (A&E)
3. Pulse oximetry, arterial blood gas, chest X-ray, echocardiography (this will confirm the diagnosis)
4. Management options include:
   ● Indomethacin (prostaglandin inhibitor) to close the PDA using medical management
   ● Surgical ligation
   ● Supportive management: oxygen, fluids, anaemia correction

7. Family tree

Candidate information

Role: You are a GP
Setting: GP surgery
Task: Data interpretation
Scenario: You see a family with an inherited disorder. The defective gene has been located on the long arm of chromosome 7. The couple are pregnant
Investigation: Family tree

Example questions

1. What do the following symbols represent?
   ◐ ■ △ ◇
2. What is the mode of inheritance?
3. What is the chance of the unborn child being affected by the condition?
4. What antenatal and postnatal screening tests are available for this condition?

Example answers

1. Carrier female, affected male, miscarriage, sex unknown
2. Autosomal recessive
3. 1 in 4 or 25%
4. Antenatal testing for cystic fibrosis: chronic villus sampling or amniocentesis.
   Postnatal testing: neonatal heel prick test or sweat test

8. Growth chart

Candidate information

Role: You are a paediatric SHO

Setting: Paediatric general outpatient clinic

Task: Data interpretation

Scenario: You see a 35-month-old boy in clinic. He has been referred by his GP due to poor weight gain. On examination you notice he has buttock wasting.

Investigation: Growth chart

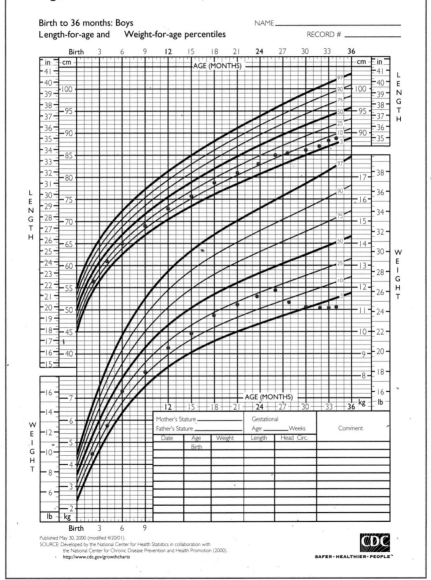

Example questions

1. What is the probable diagnosis?
2. What possibly happened at around 24 months of age?
3. What further investigations could you do?
4. How would you manage this patient?

Example answers

1. Coeliac disease
2. Introduction of wheat into the diet, such as in cereals
3. Further investigations would be:
   - Tissue transglutaminase antibodies, IgA antiendomysial antibodies, serum IgA level
   - Full blood count, iron studies, vitamin B12, bone profile
   - Stool sample
   - Endoscopy with duodenal/jejunum biopsy
4. Trial gluten-free diet

9. Urinalysis

> ### Candidate information
>
> **Role**: You are a GP
> **Setting**: GP surgery
> **Task**: Data interpretation
> **Scenario**: You see a 5-year-old girl with a history of ongoing periorbital puffiness and abdominal distension since 2 weeks
> **Investigation**: Urinalysis
>
> | | |
> |---|---|
> | Blood: | – |
> | Protein: | +++ |
> | Leucocytes: | + |
> | Nitrites: | – |
> | Glucose: | – |
> | Ketones: | – |

Example questions:

1. What is the probable diagnosis?
2. What would be your management?
3. What further investigations may be done?
4. What is the mainstay of treatment?

Example answers:

1. Nephrotic syndrome
2. Urgent referral to paediatric team

3. Full blood count (FBC), urea and electrolytes (U&E), complement levels, renal tract ultrasound, kidney biopsy
4. Prednisolone

10. EEG

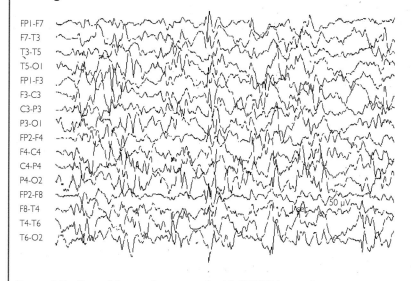

Candidate information

Role: You are a GP

Setting: GP surgery

Task: Data interpretation

Scenario: You receive a copy of the EEG result for a 10-month-old boy who you had seen with seizures. He has normal development. He is already under the paediatric neurologist

Investigation:

FP1-F7
F7-T3
T3-T5
T5-O1
FP1-F3
F3-C3
C3-P3
P3-O1
FP2-F4
F4-C4
C4-P4
P4-O2
FP2-F8
F8-T4
T4-T6
T6-O2

50 µV

From: http://emedicine.medscape.com/article/1138154-overview

Example questions:

1. What is the probable diagnosis?
2. What features of the EEG make you suspect this?
3. Which two syndromes is this patient at risk of developing?

Example answers:

1. Infantile spasm
2. Hypsarrhythmia, as demonstrated by the chaotic high-amplitude waves

3. West syndrome: triad of hysparrhythmia, infantile spasms and developmental regression/retardation, and
   - Lennox–Gastaut syndrome: can develop around 3–5 years of age and manifests with seizures (atypical absence, atonic, tonic), mental retardation and a slow spike and wave EEG pattern (<2 Hz).

Practice cases

1. Blood results

> Candidate information
>
> **Role:** You are a GP
> **Setting:** GP surgery
> **Task:** Data interpretation
> **Scenario:** You see a 10-year-old girl with a 1-year history of recurrent abdominal pain. The examination is entirely normal, and the blood results are as follows:
> **Investigation:** Blood results
>   **FBC:** Normal
>   **Liver function tests (LFTs):** Normal
>   **U&E:** Normal

Practice questions:

1. What are your differential diagnoses?
2. What investigations would you do next?
3. How would you manage this patient?

2. Stool sample

> Candidate information
>
> **Role:** You are a GP
> **Setting:** GP surgery
> **Task:** Data interpretation
> **Scenario:** You see an 8-month-girl with recurrent non-projectile vomiting. Her mother also reports intermittent episodes of loose stool. She is thriving, and examination is normal. Your colleague requested a stool sample and the result is below:
> **Investigation:** Stool sample
>   **Appearance:** Semi-formed, brown
>   **Oocytes and parasites:** Negative
>   **Helicobacter pylori:** Positive
>   **Microscopy and culture:** Negative

Practice questions:

1. What is your suspected diagnosis?
2. What further investigation could you do to confirm this?
3. How would you manage and treat this case?

3. Growth chart

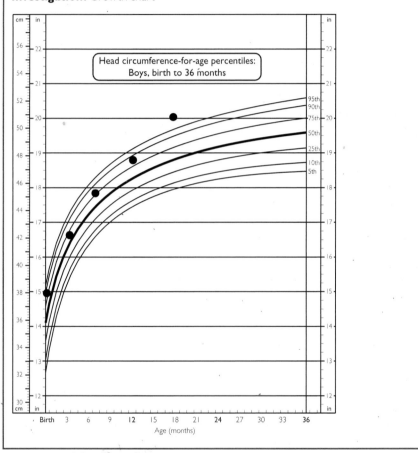

Head circumference-for-age percentiles: Boys, birth to 36 months

Practice questions

1. What are your differential diagnoses?
2. What would you do next?
3. How would you manage this patient?

Anchor statement: data interpretation

Station 3: Data interpretation		
	Expected standard **CLEAR PASS**	**PASS**
DATA INTERPRETATION	Identifies problem data Accurately interprets the data in the clinical context provided (achieves correct diagnosis)	Identifies problem data No clinical diagnosis but suggests relevant differential diagnosis
DISCUSSION	Fluent and confident in discussing management Good understanding of the evidence base (for example NICE guidelines) underpinning good paediatric practice above	Lacks confidence in discussing management Understands evidence base underpinning good paediatric practice

BARE FAIL	CLEAR FAIL	UNACCEPTABLE
Identifies problem data No clinical diagnosis or limited differential diagnosis	Fails to identify problem data Incorrect clinical diagnosis or inappropriate differential diagnosis	Fails to identify problem data Incorrect and unsafe diagnosis
Limited knowledge and understanding of management Limited understanding of evidence-based approach to paediatric practice	Poor knowledge and understanding of management Poor understanding of evidence-based approach to paediatric practice	Unreliable and unsafe response to investigations and management in paediatrics Argumentative and critical of evidence-based approach to paediatric practice

4 STRUCTURED ORAL

This station will assess your clinical knowledge and understanding of a particular child health topic. Your ability to think on your feet and discuss the topic in a clear, appropriate and professional manner will also be assessed.

Format

This 6-minute station takes place between you and the examiner. You will not be given any information prior to entering the station. Once the assessment commences, you will have 6 minutes to answer the series of questions posed by the examiner.

How to approach this station

This type of viva style of assessment, with you being directly 'interrogated' by an examiner, can be very stressful. It is important that you are focused and appear calm. Make sure you read the scenario or brief very carefully. This is important because the application of your knowledge to the specific scenario will be assessed. Before blurting out your answers, pause for a moment and think about a logical format for your answer. This is essential because you need to demonstrate to the examiner that you have sound clinical thinking and application of knowledge.

> Top tips
> - Do not be put off or disheartened by the examiner
> - Appear appropriately confident, but not overconfident or cocky
> - Ask for clarification if you do not understand the question
> - Present your answer in a logical manner
> - Do not waffle – the examiner has a list of questions to get through

Common themes

Almost any topic relevant to paediatrics could come up in this station. So it is important that you read widely. The paediatric sections of either the *Oxford Handbook of General Practice* or the *Oxford Handbook of Clinical Specialties* are useful sources of condensed information. It is also worthwhile keeping abreast of relevant National Institute of Clinical Excellence (NICE) guidelines, such as those for fever in children, urinary tract infections and head injury.

Other common themes relate to community paediatrics, child protection and health surveillance. Therefore, try to spend some time in community paediatrics. Here you may come across school nurses and their roles, the legal issues and medical issues associated with adoption and fostering, child protection issues and 'statementing'. You should also attend the child protection training run by your trust. Consider how this would apply to you if working as a GP in the community, and how you would access child health surveillance and child protection services.

Skills to demonstrate

Use the Anchor statements (pp. 68–69), reproduced with permission from the RCPCH, to understand what the examiners will be looking for. You can use it as a 'mark scheme' to grade your performance when doing the practice cases.

Worked examples and practice cases

The following worked examples highlight important paediatric areas, not covered elsewhere in this book, which may form discussion during the structured oral station, including:

- Child protection
- Special educational needs
- Paediatric public health
- Common neonatal problems
- Child development
- Paediatric emergencies
- Specific chronic disease management
- Common paediatric conditions
- Paediatric surgery

Use the practise case boxes to further develop your skills at thinking logically through a topic and succinctly discussing it.

Child protection

What constitutes child abuse?

Four categories of child abuse are recognized and these often coexist:

1. Physical abuse or non-accidental injury (NAI)
2. Emotional abuse
3. Sexual abuse
4. Neglect

A fifth category is functional or induced illness in a child instigated by a parent or guardian. The term 'Munchausen's by proxy' for this has largely fallen out of favour.

How does the Law protect children from abuse and neglect?

The following sections of The Children Act 1989/2004 are relevant:

- Section 47: provides for children at risk of significant harm (the parents may be overruled)
- Section 17: provides for children in need of assistance to flourish (it requires parental consent)

The Sexual Offences Act 2003 clarifies what is a sexual offence against a child, especially what may be classed as rape, and the Forced Marriages Act 2007 protects against forced marriages.

The Education Act 1981 provides legal guidance on education provision standards.

If you are worried that a child is at significant risk of harm, what can you do as a GP?

- Clearly communicate your concerns with appropriate members of your healthcare team, and document them clearly
- Call the appropriate child protection worker
- Be familiar with your local guidelines and your duties as a healthcare worker (www.everychildmatters.gov.uk), e.g. hospital admission may protect a child and allow a full assessment. Social services and the child protection team have a 24-hour on-call phone number
- If admission is refused, either by the parent/carer or by the admitting paediatrician, for any reason, social services can instigate a place of safety order, or the police can remove a child and place them in police protection

What if you are not sure that there is a risk?

- Check with social services whether a child or sibling is on the 'at-risk register' (this is changing, but essentially you can check if a child is known to social services)
- Check the notes of siblings and other family members for any suggestion of abuse in the past (child safety trumps confidentiality concerns here)
- Discuss with (depending on age of child) health visitor, named nurse or consultant paediatrician who is responsible for child protection in your area
- Any increase in suspicion should prompt action
- If you are still not sure, record your concerns clearly and alert other involved members of the practice team
- Review the situation every time the child is seen again in the practice

> ## Practice cases
>
> Other child protection issues you could be asked to discuss include:
>
> - Which authorities must be informed if you suspect child abuse?
> - What is the role of social services, police, school, health visitor, doctors and dentists in child protection?

Special educational needs

What causes of 'failure at school' do GPs and paediatricians encounter?

- Social problems: domestic and peer-related problems (such as bullying or sexual abuse), school absence
- School absence through illness, school refusal, truancy, neglect
- Poor home-schooling
- Educational problems: limited intellect (note that the term 'mental handicap' has been replaced by the term 'learning disability'), attention deficit hyperactivity disorder, autistic spectrum disorder, hearing or vision problems, dyslexia, dyspraxia and other physical handicaps

What legislation supports children with special educational needs?

Since the 1981 Education Act, the education authority is obliged to assess children who may need additional educational provision because of severe or complex difficulties. Following this assessment, a legally binding document is produced: the statement of special educational needs (SSEN). It is reviewed annually and is drawn up on the basis of an educational psychologist's report, medical report (from hospital and community paediatricians) and reports from other involved professionals such as therapists and a child's nursery or school. The parents are also invited to submit evidence. The child's educational needs and the provision needed to meet them are clearly outlined.

Are children with special needs looked after in special schools?

If possible, children with special educational needs are educated in mainstream schools, with extra help provided in the classroom as needed. There are special schools if mainstream education is not appropriate, and some mainstream schools have specialized language units within them. Be prepared to talk about advantages and disadvantages in types of schooling, e.g. large class sizes in state schools.

What other help is there for children with special needs?

Support may be provided by different therapists: occupational therapists, physiotherapists, speech and language therapists and classroom special needs assistants.

Parents can claim disability living allowance (DLA) for children with special needs, including a mobility component from age 5 as well as invalid care allowance (provided they are not in full-time employment). There is a care component and a mobility component to the DLA.

Practice cases

Other special educational needs issues you could be asked to discuss include:
- What do you know about dyspraxia?
- What benefits are available to children with special needs?
- Autism
- What is the role of the educational psychologist?

Paediatric public health: Example – screening

What conditions are screened for in newborn babies and why?

The following is not an exhaustive list:

- Phenylketonuria (PKU): The Guthrie test is carried out on blood on filter paper obtained by heel prick. The baby must be on full milk feeds for 3 days before testing. Untreated PKU causes severe learning disability. A low phenylalanine diet prevents the build-up of metabolites, which cause brain damage.
- Congenital hypothyroidism: Analysis of thyroxine and thyroid-stimulating hormone, also from blood on filter paper obtained by heel prick – the same sample as PKU testing. If treated early, the child grows and develops normally. Untreated it results in severe learning disability.
- Congenital cataracts: When looking through an ophthalmoscope, if white light instead of red is reflected from the retina, it suggests a cataract or other ophthalmic pathology. Immediate referral is needed and early treatment prevents permanent visual impairment.
- Cryptorchidism: If the testes in baby boys are impalpable in the scrotal sac, referral is needed. Undescended testes are at risk of infertility and malignancy. Surgery should be performed before the age of 18 months.
- Developmental dysplasia of the hip: The Barlow and Ortolani manoeuvres are carried out as part of the neonatal check and at 6 weeks; abnormal findings are confirmed by ultrasound. Early orthopaedic intervention is effective in preventing limp and painful disability from dislocated, subluxed or dysplastic hips.

- Congenital heart disease: Identification of a heart murmur is the commonest presentation. If cardiac defects at birth are missed, then irreversible cardiopulmonary changes or infective endocarditis may result.

What are important criteria for screening tests?

- The condition involved should be an important health problem
- The natural history of the disease should be known
- There should be a recognizable latent or early symptomatic phase
- There should be a test that is easy to perform and interpret
- It should be accurate, reliable, sensitive and specific
- There should be an acceptable, recognized treatment for the disease
- Treatment should be more effective if started early
- There should be a policy on who should be treated
- Diagnosis and treatment should be cost effective
- Case finding should be continuous

Paediatric public health: Example – immunization

Why do we immunize children?

In developed countries the most beneficial and cost-effective health intervention for the primary prevention of infectious diseases is immunization. One of the primary aims is to provide a population with herd immunity so that the infectious organism cannot survive by chain transmission. Effective herd immunity can only be achieved with immunization rates of around 90% of the population. This is important for the protection of those who cannot be immunized, and because no vaccine is 100% effective.

What is the current immunization schedule in the UK?

- 2 months: diphtheria/tetanus/pertussis/poliomyelitis/haemophilus type B (DTaP/IPV/Hib) (one injection) and pneumococcal vaccine (one injection)
- 3 months: DTaP/IPV/Hib (one injection) and meningococcus group C (MenC) (one injection)
- 4 months: DTaP/IPV/Hib (one injection), MenC (one injection) and pneumococcal vaccine (one injection)
- 12 months: Hib/MenC (one injection)
- 13 months: measles, mumps and rubella (MMR) (one injection) and pneumococcal vaccine (one injection)
- 3 years and 4 months–5 years: DTaP or dTaP (one injection) and MMR (one injection) (reduced dose diphtheria vaccine if aged over 10 or completed primary immunizations in infancy)
- 12–13 (girls): HPV vaccine (three injections with the second given 2 months after the first and the third given 6 months after the second)

- 13–18 years: diphtheria, tetanus and polio (Td/IPV) (one injection)

Up-to-date information on immunization and infectious disease may be found at www.immunisation.nhs.uk.

If a child is allergic to eggs, can they still have the MMR vaccine?

The MMR vaccine may contain small quantities of egg. The concern regarding serious reactions to MMR in children with egg allergy has rarely been borne out when such children have received the vaccine. The vaccine may thus be given. However, if a child has had an anaphylactic reaction to egg, it may be appropriate for the first/next dose of the vaccine to be given in hospital. This is more for parental reassurance than because of the theoretical risk of an adverse reaction. There is no good evidence that skin testing is helpful to rule out such allergies.

When should immunizations be postponed or avoided?

- Postpone immunizations if a child has a systemic febrile illness, not just 'snuffles' or 'a bit of a cough'. Taking antibiotics is not a contraindication
- Asthma and eczema are not contraindications except in the case of specific allergies (but see earlier)
- The mother being pregnant again is not a contraindication, but having an immune-compromised sibling is a contraindication to the live oral polio vaccine
- Vaccination against tuberculosis and other live vaccines should be avoided in human immunodeficiency virus (HIV)-positive children

---

Practice cases

Other paediatric public health issues you could be asked to discuss include:

- What is child health surveillance/promotion?
- What do children die from in the UK?
- Childhood obesity
- Role of the school doctor/nurse, health visitor, community midwife

---

Common neonatal problems: Example – jaundice

What causes jaundice in newborn babies? Is it common?

Jaundice is benign in most babies – it is due to problems with bilirubin metabolism and clearance. Approximately 50% of term and 80% of preterm babies become jaundiced.

When should you take notice of jaundice?

Jaundice is regarded as pathological if it occurs within 24 hours of birth or more than 3 weeks after birth. Some babies have clinically obvious jaundice for >10 days after birth. Certain risk factors (Rh incompatibility, birth trauma, infection, polycythaemia, hypothyroidism or poor feeding) may lead to high plasma bilirubin levels with a risk of neurotoxicity and kernicterus. A raised conjugated bilirubin level in a jaundiced child suggests biliary obstruction and should be referred immediately to the paediatric department. The paediatrician may refer the child on to a paediatric specialist liver unit.

Can plasma bilirubin concentration be reliably estimated by clinical examination?

No. If risk factors are present, bilirubin levels should be tested on a venous or capillary blood sample and/or transcutaneous bilirubinometry.

What is the treatment of clinically significant jaundice?

Treatment is with phototherapy with blue light. Very high levels may require an exchange transfusion.

What is breast-milk jaundice?

This is the commonest reason for jaundice lasting beyond 10 days (unconjugated hyperbilirubinaemia). Mothers can mostly be reassured that it usually resolves by 6 weeks but may continue for 3 months. The jaundice disappears if breast feeding is stopped, but this action is only advised in exceptional circumstances.

Practice cases

Other neonatal problems you could be asked to discuss include:
- Routine care at delivery and neonatal resuscitation
- Group B *Streptococcus* (GBS) in pregnancy and signs of GBS septicaemia in infancy
- Respiratory distress
- Congenital cyanotic heart disease
- Feeding problems and hypoglycaemia in infancy
- Low birth weight and prematurity
- The neonatal examination and problems that may be picked up

---

Child development: Example – flat feet in toddlers

Scenario

A mother has brought her 2-year-old daughter to the GP because she is flat footed and her feet seem to point inward a little when she runs. Whilst standing on tiptoe (which she does not do for long), there is no convincing medial arch.

How would you advise the mother?

This example serves to illustrate that anything that presents to GPs may be used in this examination. Pes planus (or flat foot) is where the arch of the foot is low. There may be valgus and eversion foot deformities. The most important advice is that flat feet are normal in children who are learning to walk. The medial arch develops over the next few years. If flat feet persist, no action is necessary provided that the medial arch of the foot restores itself on tiptoe.

The mother wants to know if there is anything that she can do to help her daughter develop healthy feet

Some research shows that children who are allowed to go barefoot until the age of 6 years have healthier feet. Some GPs suggest exercises to produce the arch; these involve the child flexing their forefoot and toes, 'like a crawly caterpillar!'

Would anything make you concerned in such a circumstance?

High arches in a small child who has a clumsy gait might raise suspicion of cerebral palsy or muscular dystrophy. Any other signs of ataxia might raise suspicion of neurological disease or a posterior fossa tumour.

> **Practice cases**
>
> Other child development issues you could be asked to discuss include:
> - Fields of child development
> - Hearing assessment
> - Normal/abnormal milestones
> - Learning difficulties
> - Communication difficulties
> - Movement disorders

Paediatric emergencies: Example – Kawasaki disease

How would you identify Kawasaki disease?

Note: You may also be given signs and symptoms of this disease in a clinical scenario. Identification is by the presence of more than five of:

KWASKI' DISEASE
IDENTIFICATION IS BY PRESENCE OF 35

- Fever for >5 days
- Bilateral non-purulent conjunctivitis
- Polymorphous rash
- Changes in lips and mouth: more reddened, dry or cracked lips
- Strawberry tongue
- Diffuse redness of oropharyngeal mucosa
- Reddened palms or soles or ulcerative oedema of the hands and feet
- Peeling of the skin on the digits of the hands and feet (convalescence)

p cervical lymphadenopathy

What are the differential diagnoses of these signs?

- Staphylococcal scalded skin syndrome
- Scarlet fever
- Drug reactions
- Stevens–Johnson syndrome
- Measles

Does a positive swab for streptococcal throat exclude Kawasaki disease?

No.

What is the management of Kawasaki disease?

- Urgently refer to hospital paediatric department
- Early treatment (<10 days) with intravenous immunoglobulin and aspirin decreases the incidence and severity of complications as well as providing symptomatic relief. Treatment may be given after this time
- Be prepared to talk about the avoidance of aspirin in young children and Reye syndrome in all cases but Kawasaki disease
- Parents should be offered support such as the Kawasaki Support Group www.patient.co.uk/leaflets/kawasaki_support_group.htm

What are the complications of Kawasaki disease?

- In the acute phase, it may cause thromboses, myocardial infarct, dysrhythmias and even death
- In the long term, scarring of coronary arteries and accelerated atherosclerosis/coronary artery disease may occur
- Coronary arteritis leading to coronary aneurysms in 20–30% of untreated patients

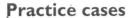

> ## Practice cases
>
> Other paediatric emergencies you could be asked
> to discuss include:
>
> - Recognition of the seriously unwell child
> - Paediatric emergencies – estimate a child's
>   weight and fluid requirement
> - Poisoning
> - Management of near-drowning
> - Management of burns
> - Sepsis or meningitis
> - Management of diabetic keto-acidosis
> - Management of severe croup, epiglottis,
>   asthma or airway obstruction
> - Management of the severely injured child

Chronic disease management: Example – paediatric asthma

What are the steps in asthma management for children?

Summary of current British Thoracic Society (BTS)/Scottish Intercollegiate
Guidelines Network (SIGN) Guidelines (revised 2011) for the management of
asthma in children:

For children aged <5 years:

- Step 1: Use an inhaled short-acting beta-agonist as needed
- Step 2: Add an inhaled steroid 200–400 µg/day or leukotriene antagonist (such
  as montelukast) if steroids are contraindicated
- Step 3: In children aged 2–5, consider a trial of montelukast and for children
  aged <2 consider step 4
- Step 4: Refer to a respiratory paediatrician

For children aged 5–12 years:

- Step 1: Use an inhaled short-acting beta-agonist as needed
- Step 2: Add an inhaled steroid 200–400 µg/day
- Step 3: Add a long-acting beta agonist (LABA). If there is a good response,
  continue LABA and increase the inhaled steroid to 400 µg/day. If there is no
  response, stop LABA, increase the inhaled steroid to 400 µg/day and consider
  a trial of montelukast or theophylline
- Step 4: Increase the inhaled steroid to 800 µg/day or equivalent
- Step 5: Add oral steroids, maintain a high-dose inhaled steroid at 800 µg/day
  and refer to a respiratory paediatrician

Up-to-date information on the BTS Asthma guidelines can be found on their
website.

Are inhaled corticosteroids safe?

Yes, if given at the recommended dose. If the dose is exceeded, then adverse effects may include adrenal suppression. There is no evidence to support preventative low-dose steroid use for episodic viral wheeze.

Which children with asthma need to be referred to a specialist clinic?

- Where there is doubt over the diagnosis
- A child who has a poor response to 800 µg/day of inhaled beclomethasone (or equivalent)
- A child who has reached stage 4 of the BTS/SIGN guideline and should be on other asthma treatments; concordance and drug delivery need careful assessment
- A child who shows a poor response to 400 µg/day of inhaled beclomethasone (or equivalent) and needs add-on therapy that the GP is unfamiliar with
- A young child <5 years old where there is uncertainty about drug delivery; this requires (at the very least) access to the expertise of a specialist asthma nurse
- A child under 1 year old; often there is doubt about the diagnosis
- Where there has been recurrent admission to hospital, which suggests a dangerous pattern of asthma (such patients are often granted 'open access' to children's assessment units or paediatric wards)
- Patients with particularly severe acute asthma, such as those needing intravenous (IV) treatment or intensive care unit (ICU) admission, should always be referred
- Where there are social factors such as neglect, abuse or poor living conditions.

Practice cases

Other chronic diseases you could be asked to discuss include:
- Diagnosis and management of childhood diabetes
- Causes and management of childhood anaemia
- Diagnosis and management of cystic fibrosis
- Childhood cancer
- Recurrent abdominal pain
- Recurrent headaches

Common paediatric conditions: Example – urinary tract infection (UTI)

You should know and be able to apply the current NICE guidelines of UTI in children. Common themes relate to the diagnosis and management of UTIs, and in particular whether or not imaging is required.

What might raise your clinical suspicion of a UTI?

- It must be considered in any small child who is septic or ill, has fever, vomiting or irritability
- It may be a cause of poor urine flow
- It may be associated with an abdominal or bladder mass
- In a verbal child, a complaint of pain on urination or abdominal pain
- Failure to thrive (consider recurrent UTI)

Would you investigate a suspected UTI before starting treatment?

Antibiotic treatment should not be delayed while awaiting results of microscopy and culture. Recent NICE guidance advocates dipping a urine sample (ideally clean catch) for nitrites and leucocytes if there are moderate symptoms and clinical suspicion (www.nice.org.uk/c6054). All children under 3 months of age with a first UTI should be referred to paediatrics or paediatric urology (depending on local referral guidelines) for assessment and further investigation. Older children with severe or recurrent UTIs should also be referred.

What further investigations might be offered and how might you explain them to an anxious parent?

Investigations to consider are ultrasound of the renal tract followed by a micturating cystourethrogram and/or a dimercaptosuccinic acid (DMSA) scan (the latter to look for renal scarring). The NICE guidelines for UTI in children have a clear recommended imaging schedule – learn it! A useful leaflet on isotope renal scans can be found on the Royal College of Radiology website (www.rcr.ac.uk/docs/patients/worddocs/radleafnmkidneyf12.doc).

You might explain the need for investigation as follows: 'Appropriate and prompt antibiotic treatment reduces the risk of kidney scarring, which can occur in children as a result of recurrent infections. Young children with urine infections (and children who have severe or recurring infections) need to have investigations done. This is to make sure that they do not have any abnormality of the kidneys, bladder or urinary tract. This is initially an ultrasound scan, which may be followed by a test called a "micturating cystourethrogram". Children with renal tract abnormalities need antibiotics to safeguard against infections and kidney damage. Children at risk of kidney scarring will be offered a further test which looks for scarring and is called a DMSA scan.'

What is the treatment for UTI?

- Empirical treatment often depends on local resistance and is usually trimethoprim or nitrofurantoin (consult the British National Formulary for children (BNFc) for the appropriate age- or weight-related dose)

- Children with renal tract abnormalities or who are awaiting further renal tract investigations should have low-dose prophylaxis (ideally with trimethoprim or nitrofurantoin – see BNFc)

Practice cases

Other common conditions you could be asked to discuss include:

- Childhood skin diseases
- Management of gastroenteritis
- Allergy in children
- Reflex anoxic seizures
- Epistaxis
- Dyspraxia
- Upper respiratory tract infections
- Differentiating minor from serious illness

Paediatric surgery: Example – pyloric stenosis

What are the clinical features of pyloric stenosis?

- Projectile vomiting – of curdled and unpleasant-smelling milk, not bile stained. The baby will be hungry and will feed immediately after vomiting
- Failure to thrive
- Dehydration
- Constipation – due to dehydration. Rabbit pellet stools
- Distended stomach, may have visible peristalsis of the stomach
- 95% have a palpable pyloric mass (like an olive) just below the right costal margin, which is more prominent after vomiting
- May have haematemesis

Are there any special investigations?

Diagnosis is based on clinical findings. A test feed may be done – the baby is given a drink, sat on the parent's lap and the examiner's hand is dipped deeply under the liver to find the 'olive-sized' pyloric thickening. A venous blood gas test in hospital may show a hypochloraemic alkalosis.

How would you manage this if it presents in A&E or general practice?

The child should be referred acutely to the hospital paediatric department for assessment, metabolic stabilization and subsequent transfer to the care of a paediatric surgeon. The operation performed is a pyloromyotomy.

What is the epidemiology of pyloric stenosis?

This condition usually develops in the first 3–6 weeks of life, and rarely presents in infants over the age of 12 weeks. It is commonest in first-born, male children.

Practice cases

Other paediatric surgical conditions you could be asked to discuss include:

- Appendicitis
- Abdominal wall hernias
- Neck lumps
- Transplant patients
- Intussusception – recognition and management
- Circumcision and urological problems
- Congenital abnormalities requiring urgent referral

Anchor statement: structured oral

Station 4: Structured oral		
	Expected standard **CLEAR PASS**	**PASS**
DISCUSSION	Knowledge and its application in clinical setting Considers ethical issues Clear, appropriate and professional	Able to solve problems Reasonable clinical thinking

© Royal College of Paediatrics and Child Health 2012, reproduced with permission.

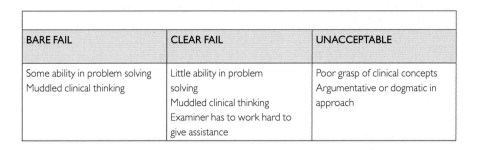

BARE FAIL	CLEAR FAIL	UNACCEPTABLE
Some ability in problem solving Muddled clinical thinking	Little ability in problem solving Muddled clinical thinking Examiner has to work hard to give assistance	Poor grasp of clinical concepts Argumentative or dogmatic in approach

5

CLINICAL ASSESSMENT

Your examination and clinical assessment of a child or adolescent gives essential information about the possible diagnosis. This station will not only assess your ability to fluently perform the correct clinical examination, but also assesses your clinical acumen in detecting and interpreting the clinical signs.

Format

You will be given the brief once you have entered the station and been instructed by the examiner of which clinical examination to conduct. The examiner will introduce you to the child and parent/carer. You will have 9 minutes to perform your clinical examination *and* answer the examiner's questions. The examiner is at liberty to intervene at any time during the station, and will enquire about the clinical findings, your interpretation and management of the case.

How to approach this station

Always introduce yourself to the parent/carer and child, and establish a rapport. This is important, because it can help make an anxious child feel at ease if they observe you interacting with the parent first. Ask for permission from the parent to conduct the required clinical examination. Ensure that you wash your hands between cases and remember to treat each child with courtesy and dignity. Always remember to ask for the parents' and child's permission before undressing the child, and always ask the child if he or she has any pain anywhere before starting the examination.

You must listen carefully to the instructions given to you by the examiner. For example, you may be asked to only perform a specific part of the cardiovascular examination such as 'examine the praecordium' or 'examine the peripheral pulses' rather than 'examine the cardiovascular system'. If you are uncertain about where to start, then ask for clarification because failure to carry out the correct task will cost you valuable time and marks.

You should demonstrate an empathetic approach and help the child feel at ease throughout the station. You should also aim to maintain a good rapport with the parent. If you feel comfortable to report your findings to the examiner as you go along then you can do so. The examiner can interrupt you to ask questions at any stage during the station – do not be put off by this. It is important that you are able to correctly detect and interpret the clinical signs, offer differential diagnosis and suggest an appropriate management plan.

It is vital that you have a structured approach to the clinical examinations and that you can perform the examination with confidence. Remember, practise makes perfect – so make sure you practise a lot.

Dealing with a shy, frightened or crying child

Firstly, don't panic! Secondly, don't think you will automatically fail! Then acknowledge that these things happen and allow the child and parent some time together. Gradually begin to interact with the child, and generate trust and their cooperation. Pre-verbal children often respond to interesting sights and sounds such as a shiny bunch of keys, a rattle or bubbles. Be inventive with what you have available. Attempt to distract them if possible, e.g. by offering to let them hold a toy, playing 'peep-oh' or pulling faces. Let them play with any equipment you may have, providing it is safe. Older (verbal) children can be challenged: 'I bet you can't open your mouth as wide as mine,' or involved in the examination, i.e. 'What sound does your tummy make?'

If a child is clearly distressed, you may need to give them more time to calm down and the station may need to be deferred. Examiners will make allowance for this. Always remember the child comes first, and he or she must be treated with understanding and respect.

Common themes

Technically *any* clinical examination could be tested in this station, however the key systems examinations likely to come up include:

- Cardiovascular
- Respiratory
- Abdominal
- Neurological
- Surgical
- Other, e.g. endocrine, skin, eye

Skills to demonstrate

Use the Anchor statements (pp. 98–99), reproduced with permission from the RCPCH, to understand what the examiners will be looking for. You can use it as a 'mark scheme' to grade your performance when doing the practise cases.

Examples of full systems examinations

The rest of this chapter outlines the key systems examinations likely to be tested in this station. Details about important paediatric topics have also been included to aid your revision.

The most important advice to reinforce is the need to listen to the examiner's instructions. They may give you a general or specific task to carry out, and you must act accordingly or be at risk of losing marks.

Cardiovascular examination

Remember: Inspection, Percussion, Palpation, Auscultation

Inspection

- Look at nutritional status – is the child especially small, thin or fat?
- Consider dysmorphic features, which may suggest a syndrome, e.g. Down, Marfan, Turner or Noonan syndromes
- Check for cyanosis:
  - peripheral, e.g. nail beds
  - central, e.g. under tongue
- Check for pallor – anaemia (conjunctiva/mucous membranes)
- Check for plethora – polycythaemia (cyanotic heart disease)
- Check for surgical scars (Figure 5.1) (ensure that you examine the back and under the arms):
  - left thoracotomy, e.g. patent ductus arteriosus (PDA) ligation, aortic coarctation repair, pulmonary artery banding
  - sternotomy, e.g. complex cardiac surgery
- Fingers:
  - check clubbing, e.g. cyanotic heart disease
  - splinter haemorrhages, e.g. subacute bacterial endocarditis
  - tendon xanthoma, e.g. dyslipidaemia
- Hands:
  - absent radii (VACTERL, a non-random association of abnormalities that may be associated with statin use in the first trimester of pregnancy: Vertebral anomalies, Anal atresia, Cardiac defect, TracheoEsophageal fistula, Renal, Limb abnormalities)
  - absent thumbs (Holt–Oram syndrome – about 75% have heart problems; all have at least one limb abnormality that affects bones in the wrist).

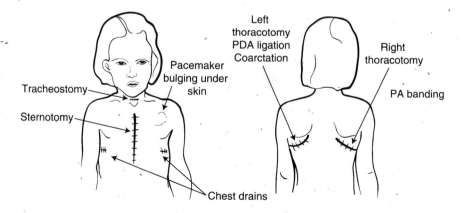

FIGURE 5.1 Surgical scars in children who have had heart or lung surgery.

Percussion

Percussion is not often helpful but it may be useful in pericardial effusion. The liver edge may be percussed for hepatomegaly in cardiac failure.

Palpation

- **General**
  - check both radial and brachial pulses (brachial is often easier to feel)
  - causes of absent brachial/radial pulses:
- congenital absence
- previous cardiac surgery, e.g. coarctation of the aorta
- angioplasty
- absent/delayed femoral pulse – coarctation
- **Heart rate**
  - bradycardia – congenital/complete heart block/beta-blockers
  - tachycardia – anxiety, thyrotoxicosis
- **Rhythm**
  - sinus arrhythmia (pulse rate decreases on inspiration – a normal finding that is more pronounced in sporty children)
  - irregular: atrial fibrillation (AF) and ectopics (exercise abolishes these)
- **Volume**
  - decreased volume: shock/hypovolaemia, heart failure or aortic stenosis
  - increased volume (high output states): anaemia, thyrotoxicosis and CO_2 retention
- **Character** (felt at the carotid in the older child or at the brachial artery in the younger child):
  - slowly rising pulse –aortic stenosis (AS)
  - collapsing pulse – aortic incompetence (AI)
  - pulsus paradoxus seen in acute asthma and pericardial effusion (very unlikely to be seen in the exam, which uses clinically stable children with clinically stable signs)
  - jerky pulse – hypertrophic cardiomyopathy (HCM)

A femoral pulse that is absent/delayed = coarctation of the aorta.

Ask to check the blood pressure (BP). For the cuff to be an appropriate size it must occlude two-thirds of the upper arm. Refer to centile charts for age-appropriate values.

- **Apex beat position.** In the fourth to fifth intercostal space inside the mid-clavicular line (MCL), displacement to the left suggests cardiomegaly or spinal abnormality, e.g. scoliosis/pectus excavatum. Dextrocardia is where the apex beat is felt on the right side, e.g. Kartagener syndrome, which is characterized by transposition of the internal organs of the body as well as congenital malformation of respiratory cilia with resulting sinusitis and bronchiectasis. Therefore, if you cannot feel an apex beat, always check on the opposite side.
- **Thrills**
  - Left parasternal = right ventricular hypertrophy
  - Lower left sternal edge = ventricular septal defect

- Upper left sternal edge = pulmonary stenosis
- Suprasternal = aortic stenosis
- **Type**
  - Forceful = left ventricular hypertrophy
  - Heave = right ventricular hypertrophy (parasternal left sternal border)

Auscultation

Unless instructed otherwise by the examiner, examine all four areas (Figure 5.2):

1. Aortic – right second intercostal space (ICS)
2. Pulmonary – left second ICS
3. Tricuspid – left lower sternal edge
4. Mitral – left fifth ICS, mid-clavicular line
   - **Hearts sounds**
     - Murmurs
     - Added sounds
     - First heart sound – closure of mitral and tricuspid valves
     - Second heart sound – closure of aortic and pulmonary valves. Note physiological split of second heart sound that widens on inspiration. Remember a fixed split-second heart sound = atrial septal defect (ASD).
   - **Murmurs**
     - Loudness is graded 1–6 systolic and 1–4 diastolic
     - A palpable thrill represents a murmur >Grade 4
     - Site
     - Radiation
     - Timing, e.g. continuous murmur (machinery) in PDA
     - Pitch
     - Relationship to posture and respiration

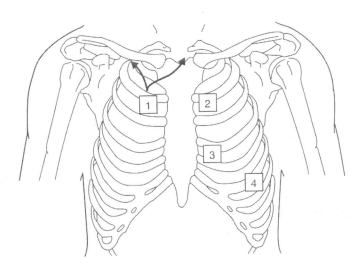

FIGURE 5.2   Auscultation areas.

Chapter 5 Clinical assessment

- **Innocent murmur (benign)**
  - no symptoms
  - systolic
  - short
  - soft
  - normal split P2 (widens on inspiration)
  - varies with posture
  - normal ECG, chest X-ray and echocardiogram
- **Normal murmurs**
  - benign (see earlier)
  - pulmonary flow – best heard at L second ICS
  - venous hum – best heard above clavicle
  - neonatal peripheral pulmonary artery stenosis
- **Pathological murmurs (systolic)**
  - ventricular septal defect – lower left sternal edge
  - pulmonary stenosis – upper left sternal edge
  - atrial septal defect – upper left sternal edge, fixed split P2
  - aortic stenosis – second right upper ICS (possible bicuspid aortic valve)
  - coarctation of the aorta – systolic murmur radiating to the back
  - mitral incompetence – mitral area
  - mitral valve prolapse – mitral area

Cardiovascular cases

The following cases could be tested:

Cyanotic congenital heart disease

One-third of congenital cardiac defects:

- Transposition of great vessels
- Fallot tetralogy
- Pulmonary atresia
- Shunt R to L

These children are far more likely to be seen in an examination post operation, on the basis that clinically unstable children will not be used in OSCEs.

Acyanotic congenital heart disease

Two-thirds of congenital cardiac defects are:

- Ventral septal defect (VSD)
- Atrial septal defect (ASD)
- Patent ductus arteriosus (PDA)
- Pulmonary stenosis (PS)
- Aortic stenosis (AS)
- Coarctation
- Shunt left to right

Respiratory examination

It is extremely important to listen to the examiner's instructions. Only undress the child to the waist after asking the parents' and child's permission. This is particularly important with adolescent girls.

Remember: Inspection, Percussion, Palpation, Auscultation.

Inspection

- General nutritional status .
- Check for respiratory aids and devices, e.g. spacers, peak flow, supplemental oxygen
- Check for clubbing (cystic fibrosis, congenital cyanotic heart disease)
- Check for cyanosis (respiratory and cardiac causes)
- Listen for stridor, both inspiratory and expiratory, and wheeze
- Check skin, e.g. eczema, or possibility of asthma/atopy
- **Chest shape**
  - Deformity, e.g. scoliosis
  - Asymmetry, e.g. fibrosis/hypoplasia
  - Hyperinflation, e.g. asthma
  - Harrison's sulcus – association with chronic respiratory distress (surgery may reverse this sign)
  - Absent pectoralis major – Poland syndrome (an absent or underdeveloped pectoralis on one side of the body and webbing of the fingers of the ipsilateral hand)
  - Pectus excavatum (hollow chest)
  - Pectus carinatum (pigeon chest)
- **Chest scars:** Such as chest drain scars or a tracheostomy scar (see Figure 5.1).
  - Accessory muscles
  - Nasal flaring, intercostal or subcostal recession
  - Use of abdominal muscles
- **Respiratory rate**
  - Infant: 20–40/min
  - 5-year-old: 15–25/min
  - 10-year-old: 15–20/min
- **Cough**
  - Barking = laryngeal
  - Moist = lower respiratory tract infection
  - Paroxysmal = pertussis

Palpation

- Check the position of the trachea – deviation with effusion and pneumothorax
- Check chest expansion by circling hands around the child's chest, placing thumbs at level of the nipples – is it symmetrical or reduced? (>4 cm is normal)

- **Tactile vocal fremitus (TVF):** Place the palm of the hand on the upper chest wall and ask the child to say '99', comparing left to right. Increased TVF occurs in consolidation and is reduced or absent with collapse and/or pleural thickening and/or effusion.

Percussion

This is useful to assess the presence of hyperinflation, i.e. with increased resonance, to check liver size or determine presence of consolidation, effusion or collapsed lung.

- Resonant – normal
- Hyperresonant – pneumothorax
- Dull – consolidation and fibrosis
- Stony dull – pleural effusion

Auscultation

- **Normal:** vesicular sounds
- **Abnormal:**
  - **bronchial:** harsh sounds, expiratory phase same length as inspiration
  - **breaths diminished or absent:** suggest no air or fluid
  - **expiratory wheeze:** asthma/bronchiolitis/foreign body
  - **fine crepitations:** fibrosis/pulmonary oedema
  - **coarse crepitations:** infective/bronchiectasis
  - **pleural rub:** only with dry pleurisy, lost with effusion.
- **Vocal resonance**
  - Ask the child to say '99' whilst listening over both lung fields
  - Increased with consolidation
  - Lost or reduced with fluid/no air
  - Listen for whispering pectoriloquy or aegophony, which can be heard just above a pleural effusion.

Abdominal examination

Introduce yourself to the parents and child and remember to ask permission to examine the child. Modesty must be observed using a blanket. Remember warm hands are helpful for examination.

Listen to the instructions from the examiner and only carry out what is asked of you, e.g. 'Please examine for a spleen' or 'Please examine the abdomen'.

Remember: Inspection, Percussion, Palpation, Auscultation

Check for:

- **Face and mucous membrane:** anaemia (mucous membranes), jaundice (sclera), spider naevi, mouth for pigmentation – Peutz–Jeghers/Addison or angioma (hereditary haemorrhagic telangiectasia)
- **Dysmorphic features:** mucopolysaccharidoses
- **Chronic liver disease:** stigmata – palmar erythema, clubbing, leuconychia, koilonychia
- **Tongue:** Down (pseudomacroglossia), Beckwith–Wiedemann (macroglossia)

The causes of clubbing in children are:
- – Cystic fibrosis (CF)
- – Inflammatory bowel disease (Crohn disease/colitis)
- – Congenital cyanotic heart disease

Abdominal inspection

You should search for scars, e.g. stoma (ileostomy/colostomy), splenectomy/appendicectomy, major surgery, laparoscopy (Figure 5.3). Striae may be present. A hernia may be visible in the abdominal wall or as a mass on inspection of the scrotum, e.g. hydrocoele and hernia.

- ● **Abdominal distension**
  - – Fat
  - – Faeces – constipation/Hirschsprung
  - – Flatus – aerophagy/malabsorption
  - – Fluid – ascites
  - – 'Flipping big mass' or fetus (it is highly unlikely that a pregnant child would consent to be a DCH examination patient but be aware that this is a possibility in practice).

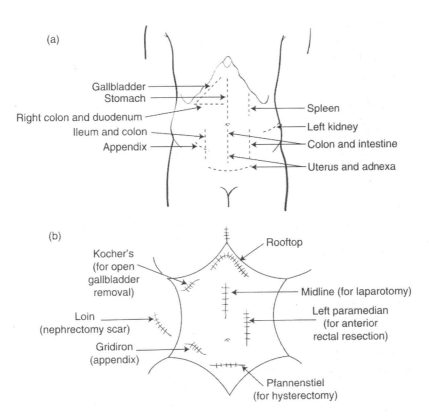

FIGURE 5.3 (a) Abdominal scar identification. (b) Abdominal incisions and their names..

Palpation

First explain to the child and parent what you are going to do, and be very gentle. Examination consists of both superficial and deep palpation of all four quadrants in turn. If tenderness is elicited, try to localize it and check for guarding or rebound. Watch the child's face at all times for any sign of discomfort. Distract younger children with comments such as, 'Can we feel lunch in your tummy?'

- **Individual organs**
  - **Liver** – start the examination in the right iliac fossa (RIF) and work up towards the right costal margin. A palpable liver in children is not unusual up to 2 cm. Percuss the upper border of the liver as well as the lower to exclude hyperinflation as a cause of hepatomegaly.
  - **Spleen** – start the examination in the RIF and work up towards the left upper quadrant. To feel the spleen you may need to turn the child onto their right side and ask them to take a deep breath. Feel for the splenic notch. This is not a consistent finding in children.
  - **Kidney** – examine bimanually in order to palpate for a kidney. An enlarged kidney may be ballotable.
- **Abdominal masses**

Try to identify site, size and consistency. Check for mobility and tenderness.

Percussion/auscultation

- Fluid, i.e. ascites – test for shifting dullness
- Mass/organomegaly
- Bowel sounds
- Renal bruits (in neurofibromatosis may have hypertension due to renal artery stenosis)
- Testes – do not routinely examine; only if requested by examiner

Lastly, 'I would like to conclude my examination by…'

- Examining the external genitalia
- Plotting height and weight on a growth chart
- Dipping the urine for blood, protein, leucocytes, nitrites, and glucose

Thyroid examination

Remember: Inspection, Percussion, Palpation, Auscultation

Inspection

Look for goitre and also examine the neck for a thyroglossal cyst (protrusion of tongue causes cyst to move). Also look for ectopic thyroid (back of tongue). Take this opportunity to also assess the thyroid status (see Table 5.1).

Percussion

Percuss to assess for any retrosternal extension.

Table 5.1 **Clinical features of hypothyroidism and hyperthyroidism**

Hypothyroidism	Hyperthyroidism
Obesity	Sweating
Short stature	Increased appetite
Puffy eyes	Weight loss
Dry skin	Goitre and/or bruit
Slow pulse	Fine tremor
Cold intolerance	Warm moist palms
Delayed relaxation of tendon reflexes	Exophthalmos
	Lid lag and lid retraction
	Ophthalmoplegia
	CVS – high output state, ejection systolic murmur, hypertension
	Proximal myopathy

Palpation

Examine the patient from behind to feel the neck; swallowing with water will help. Remember a retrosternal thyroid may cause palpable tracheal deviation in the suprasternal notch.

Auscultation

Listen to assess for any bruits. Bear in mind the other causes of neck lumps.

Neurological examination

Perform a relevant neurological examination and then look at the associated features. Use a holistic approach and observe the whole scene, considering mobility aids, nutrition and other impairments such as hearing and vision. Practise your approach to examining a child in a wheelchair so that you appear confident in the examination. *Never* make assumptions about a child's mobility or intellectual ability from their appearance.

Sometimes the examiner will direct you to ask some initial questions. It is important to direct these to both the child and the parent, and to include those about the child's schooling.

General approach

Introduce yourself to the child and parent and ask the permission of both to examine the child. Put the child at ease – chatting to them will also give you an idea of speech problems/learning difficulties.

- ● **Observation**
  - – Posture/limb alignment
  - – Wheelchair/specialist seating

- Splints
- Shoe raises
- Any obvious abnormalities with limbs/dysmorphic features
- **Gait abnormalities**
  - Hemiplegia – if walking, try to elicit more subtle signs of a hemiplegia by asking the child to run or distracting them (e.g. by asking them to count backwards whilst walking)
  - Spastic scissoring gait
  - Ataxia
  - Proximal weakness/waddling gait – to elicit proximal weakness ask the child to stand from sitting in a chair with their arms folded or try to elicit Gower sign (Figure 5.4). If the patient is Gower positive, they will not be able to stand from lying on their back without using their hands – they tend to roll over then walk their hands up their legs

Relevant examination

- **Neurological**
  - inspection of limbs – scars, contractures, muscle wasting
  - test limbs in an age appropriate way with clear instructions to the child – tone, power, reflexes, coordination, sensation, proprioception
  - examine the back for scars, scoliosis or evidence of spina bifida
  - look at the feet/shoes

- **Sensory**
  - hearing – is there a need for hearing aids?
  - vision – is the patient wearing glasses?
  - squint
  - speech and language, including dentistry/oral care

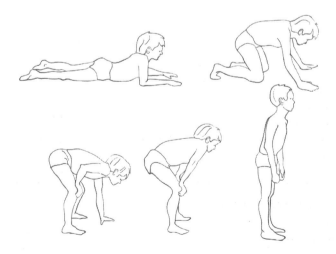

FIGURE 5.4   Gower sign (seen in Duchenne muscular dystrophy).

- **Schooling – statemented?** What support does the child have in school? (For information on the statement of special educational needs, see Chapter 4)
- **Diet**
  - swallowing OK?
  - hyoscine patch for secretions?
  - percutaneous endoscopic gastrostomy (PEG)
- **Any other medical problems**

Approach to examining a child in a wheelchair

- Introduce yourself to the child and parent
- Put them at ease
- Ask permission from the child and parent
- Observe
- Ask what the child can do – they may always be in a wheelchair but are able to move their arms and legs, or they may just use the wheelchair for trips out of the house and have a different way of moving around in the home. Find out if they can move to the couch to be examined.

Much of the examination relies on good observation, however it is possible to examine the patient's limbs while they are in a wheelchair. Practise this so that you are not thrown in the examination if the child is not on the couch:

- Start by observing the limbs, their position/posture, abnormal/involuntary movements
- Look for any splints
- Examine the patient for scars and ask the child/parent if there are any hidden scars – for example, scars from surgery to the tendo-achilles may be covered by socks
- Sit the child forward and look at their back for scars/scoliosis/evidence of spina bifida

Examine the limbs as far as possible:

- Inspection – wasting, contractures, scars, fasciculations
- Tone
- Power
- Reflexes
- Coordination
- Sensation
- In addition, look at the range of movement of the joints (passive and active) and look for contractures

If asked to continue, other relevant parts of the examination may include:

- Looking for hyoscine patches
- Examining PEG site
- Listening to lungs
- Assessing for squint
- Head – circumference, fontanelles, shunts

Common neurological cases

Cerebral palsy

Cerebral palsy is a non-progressive motor disorder caused by brain disease.
Look for the following upon inspection:

- Wheelchair
- Braces
- Calipers
- Leg/arm splints (ankle foot orthoses)
- Shoe raises
- Pressure care
- Spine abnormality
- Size and shape of skull and fontanelles (microcephaly?, hydrocephalus?)
- Face
- Any trouble with swallowing/excessive saliva? (for which they may be wearing a hyoscine patch)
- Hearing aids
- Glasses
- Squint
- Feeding tubes

Limbs

- Posture
- Ability to sit unaided
- Abnormal movements
- Scars/contractures, e.g. shortened Achilles' tendons
- Tone – increased (clonus – best tested at the ankle; the patient may also have clasp knife spasticity)
- Power – may be decreased
- Reflexes – may be increased
- Sensation – normal
- May have extensor plantars
- Coordination – may have ataxia or reduced control due to weakness

Gait

- Try to elicit subtle weakness by requesting manoeuvres that make it more obvious:
  - running, heel-to-toe walking and walking on tip-toes
  - distracting the child by asking them to recite their address or count backwards whilst walking
- May have a stiff-legged, 'scissored' gait
- May have a broad-based ataxic gait
- May have a stiff leg that is swung round
- Look at the upper limbs when they are walking. Is there a loss of natural arm swing, one arm flexed, hand making a fist?

Cerebral palsy in a small child

- Look for hand preference – babies should not show hand preference before the age of 1 year
- Look for scissoring of the legs when the child is lying on their back/lifted

Describe the pattern of neurology you find:

- Hemiplegia
- Quadriplegia
- Diplegia
- Monoplegia
- Ataxia
- Athetoid/dyskinetic
- Spastic

What other medical problems may the child have?

- Deafness
- Visual problems
- Epilepsy
- Contractures
- Dislocation of the hip
- Scoliosis
- Poor lung function/recurrent chest infections
- Poor coordination/ataxia
- Swallowing difficulties
- Reflux
- Nutritional deficiency
- Pooling of saliva/poor dentition
- Learning disabilities
- Incontinence
- Constipation
- Problems with pressure areas

The child with **multiple problems** should be managed by a multidisciplinary team. The team may include:

- Community paediatrician
- GP
- Physiotherapist
- Occupational therapist
- Speech therapist
- Dietician
- Gastroenterologist
- Orthopaedic surgeon
- Neurologist

Other considerations include:

- Support groups, e.g. www.cerebralpalsyinfo.org and www.scope.org.uk

- Education
- Respite care
- Benefits and financial support
- Mobility aids
- Management of hearing and vision problems

The types of cerebral palsy are as follows:

- **Quadriplegia** – all four limbs affected
- **Hemiplegia** – involvement of the right or left arm and leg
- **Diplegia** – involvement of both legs more than the arms

These may be:

- **Spastic** – increased tone that may affect most movements, or just a particular muscle group or limb. Although the initial insult does not progress, the spasticity may worsen with time. Spastic cerebral palsy results from damage to the motor area of the cerebral cortex
- **Ataxic** – poor coordination, hypotonia, tremor and other cerebellar signs, such as nystagmus. Truncal ataxia and a wide-based gait may be observed. Ataxic cerebral palsy results from damage to the cerebellum
- **Dyskinetic/athetoid** – athetosis describes the constant writhing movements that result from a lack of control of movement. These children may also have difficulty with their speech caused by damage to the basal ganglia
- **Mixed picture**

What is the aetiology?

Cerebral palsy is caused by prenatal, perinatal or postnatal damage to the developing brain (most cases are thought to be due to an insult in utero). The damage to the developing brain, e.g. the motor cortex, is a one-off insult and does not progress or worsen with time. The signs and symptoms, however, may appear to evolve as the child fails to meet their milestones of increasingly complex motor tasks and as the spasticity may worsen with time.

Causes include:

- **Prenatal**
  - developmental brain abnormalities
  - IUGR
  - prematurity – more common in very premature babies
  - congenital infection
- **Perinatal**
  - asphyxia at birth
  - ischaemia, e.g. placental abruption
  - trauma, e.g. forceps delivery
- **Postnatal insults to the still developing brain**
  - severe infection such as encephalitis/meningitis/cerebral abscess
  - hypoxic brain injury

- kernicterus – unconjugated bilirubin (fat soluble) can cross the blood–brain barrier and cause damage to the basal ganglia. Less common now through the careful monitoring of bilirubin levels, exchange transfusions and the decreased incidence of haemolytic disease of the newborn
- trauma
- stroke/intracranial haemorrhage
- recurrent seizures/status epilepticus
- severe prolonged hypoglycaemia.

Further information and support can be found on www.cerebralpalsyinfo.org and www.scope.org.uk.

Down syndrome (trisomy 21)

What to look for on examination (Figure 5.5)

Examining a child with an appearance suggestive of Down syndrome

- Introduce yourself and seek permission from parent and child to examine
- Stand back and sensitively comment on the patient's short stature/facial characteristics
- Examine the hands

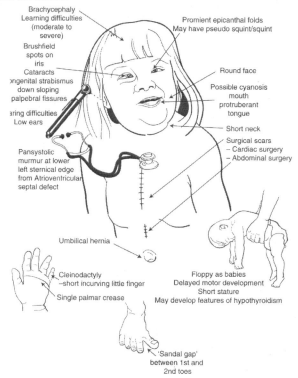

FIGURE 5.5   Features of Down syndrome.

- Conduct cardiovascular examination
- Conduct abdominal examination
- Conduct motor and development examination
- Test hearing and vision

What medical problems may the child have?

- Hearing loss – increased incidence of glue ear (conductive hearing loss) and sensorineural hearing loss
- Hypothyroidism
- Cardiac defects – especially atrioventricular septal defect (AVSD)
- Duodenal atresia
- Umbilical hernia
- Early-onset Alzheimer disease
- Cataract
- Atlantoaxial instability
- Leukaemia
- Males: infertility
- Females: delayed menarche

How would you manage a child with trisomy 21 in your practice?

- **General**: multidisciplinary team, child-centred care
- **Medically**: monitoring for hypothyroidism, prompt treatment of infections (upper respiratory/ears), monitoring of cardiac disease
- **Surgically** – referral for correction of cardiac defects, duodenal atresia, hernia repair, grommets for glue ear
- **Schooling** – almost all children will have special educational needs and will have a 'Statement of Special Educational Needs'. The degree of extra support needed is very variable
- **Other issues** – genetic counselling, family counselling and support (support groups such as www.downs-syndrome.org.uk)

Genetic counselling – Down syndrome

The family want another baby. How would you counsel them about the risks?

Explain that most cases of Down syndrome arise during early in the development of the baby, when the cells are dividing. Sometimes the chromosomes (which contain genes) are not split evenly and by chance the baby gets three copies instead of two copies of a particular chromosome (21). Mostly this is a chance event (95% – non-disjunction during meiosis). However, occasionally one of the parents can carry a faulty copy of a gene (5% of cases; Robertsonian translocation). In these cases the risk of recurrence is higher and both parents should have their chromosomes looked at (karyotyping) to detect this.

The risk of having a child with Down syndrome increases with maternal age as cell division is more likely to be faulty in the older mother. However, due to the larger number of young women giving birth, the majority of babies with trisomy 21 are born to young mothers. The background risk for all ages is 1 in 650.

Tests can be offered to screen for Down syndrome in future pregnancies, including an early scan (nuchal thickness scans) and triple testing (a blood test). These can give an idea of risk but will not indicate whether the baby is definitely affected. Higher risk mothers can go on to have more definitive testing, where a sample of cells is collected either by amniocentesis (where a small amount of amniotic fluid from around the baby is collected via a thin needle) or chorionic villus sampling (where a few cells are collected from the placenta). All tests can give false results. The invasive tests do carry a small risk of miscarriage and infection.

Breaking news that you feel a baby may have Down syndrome

Further information and support can be found at www.downs-syndrome.org.uk.

Tuberous sclerosis

What to look for on examination

- Look at the skin:
  - periungual/subungual fibromas
  - adenoma sebaceum
  - hypomelanotic macules/ash leaf-shaped depigmented patches (which fluoresce under Wood light)
  - shagreen patch over lumbar spine
- Look for evidence of epilepsy – alert bracelet? gum hypertrophy – phenytoin?
- Look for evidence of renal/cardiac problems – can get renal cysts and tumours such as angiomyolipomas and cardiac rhabdomyomata
- Look for problems with eyesight – can get tumours affecting the eyes, e.g. retinal phakomata
- May also get cerebral astrocytomas

What medical problems may the child have?

- Epilepsy/infantile spasms
- Learning difficulties/developmental delay
- Problems relating to tumours in cardiac, renal and CNS systems, and on retina
- Mostly benign tumours but some malignant potential

How would you investigate a child with tuberous sclerosis?

- Examination of the skin with a Wood lamp
- Ophthalmological examination

- May need imaging such as a renal ultrasound (US), magnetic resonance imaging (MRI) brain
- May need epilepsy investigations such as an electroencephalogram (EEG)/MRI
- Plot on growth chart
- Screen family
- Genetic testing sometimes used

What sort of management might they need?

- Multidisciplinary team
- Genetics
- Neurology/neurosurgery
- Ophthalmology
- Dermatology/plastics
- Other medical specialities such as cardiology/renal
- Support with learning difficulties – statementing
- Support with epilepsy – education, monitoring, etc.
- Family screening, support and consideration of antenatal testing

Information and support groups for affected families such as the Tuberous Sclerosis Association at www.tuberous-sclerosis.org

What do you know about the inheritance?

Autosomal dominant (20%) or spontaneous mutation (80%).

Duchenne muscular dystrophy

What to look for on examination

- **General inspection**:
  - wheelchair (by 12 years most children are unable to walk)
  - look for scoliosis
  - look for scars/muscle contractures
  - pseudohypertrophy of calves
- If younger (onset 1–4 years):
  - gait – waddling gait
  - muscle weakness. Positive Gower sign – ask the child to lie on the floor and stand up. They will tend to walk their hands up their legs due to proximal weakness (see Figure 5.4)

On examination, there will be muscle weakness and the child may have learning difficulties. If there is time, consider examining respiratory and cardiovascular systems for:

- Cardiomyopathy
- Respiratory weakness

How would you investigate a child with possible muscular dystrophy?

- Raised serum creatine kinase
- Electromyogram (EMG) studies
- Muscle biopsy – abnormal dystrophin
- Genetic testing

What do you know about the inheritance?

- X-linked recessive inheritance – screen other children in the family by testing their creatine kinase levels
- Can offer prenatal testing – chorionic villus sampling (CVS)
- Incidence 1/3000 male live births

Becker muscular dystrophy

This is a milder form of muscular dystrophy similar to Duchenne, which tends to present later, when the child is about 10–12 years old. Survival is usually to middle age.

How would you manage a child with Becker muscular dystrophy?

- Physiotherapy, mobility aids, stretches and splinting to avoid contractures
- Management of scoliosis
- Respiratory support
- Family support and education (e.g. www.muscular-dystrophy.org)
- Family screening/antenatal diagnosis/genetic counselling

Neurofibromatosis

What to look for on examination

- Look at the skin
  - axillary freckling
  - café au lait spots. Light brown patches on the skin (>5 mm in children, >15 mm in adults/adolescents)
  - neurofibromas
- Look at the eyes:
  - Lisch nodules/iris hamartomas
  - optic glioma
- Look for a hearing aid
- Examine the back for scoliosis
- Offer to check the BP – can have phaeochromocytoma (tumour of adrenal medulla) or renal artery stenosis
- Look at relatives – does the mother have similar skin lesions?

Type I

- >6 café au lait spots
- Axillary freckling
- Nodular neurofibromata (after puberty)
- Other features include learning disabilities and epilepsy

Type 2

- Bilateral acoustic neuroma
- Deafness
- Cerebellopontine angle tumour
- Associated features include hypertension due to renal artery stenosis and phaeochromocytoma, rarely sarcomatous change

What do you know about the inheritance?

Type 1 (the gene is found on chromosome 17) and type 2 (on chromosome 22). Inheritance is autosomal dominant or it may arise from a spontaneous mutation. If there is a known mutation in the family, then antenatal testing can be offered.

What treatment is available?

Treatment is aimed at alleviating symptoms, particularly pressure symptoms of tumours on nerves, bone and in the brain. This may involve surgery. Occasionally tumours can become malignant and chemotherapy or radiotherapy may be needed. MRI scans can detect lesions such as acoustic neuromas when they are very small so that they can be removed early.

Further information and support can be found at: www.nfauk.org.

Cerebellar examination

A disturbance of cerebellar function leads to a lack of coordination of movement. The following signs are indicative of cerebellar dysfunction:

- Scanning dysarthria
- Nystagmus
- Dysdiadochokinesis
- Intention tremor
- Past pointing dysmetria
- Ataxic gait (poor heel-to-toe walking)
- Romberg sign, a tendency to sway or fall while standing upright with the feet together. This usually indicates an inner ear problem or a failure of proprioception

Gait

- **Normal variations**
  - toe walking (tiptoeing) – 'little ballerina syndrome'. This may also be an early indicator of myopathy and spastic diplegia (cerebral palsy)
  - in-toeing and out-toeing
  - bow legs (Genu varum)
  - knock knees (Genu valgum). Pathological causes include rickets and Blount disease

- **Abnormal gaits** (Figure 5.6):
  - broad-based gait is often associated with cerebral palsy
  - waddling gait is often associated with untreated developmental dysplasia of the hip and Duchenne muscular dystrophy
  - hemiplegic gait
  - spastic diplegia
  - ataxic gait (cerebellar dysfunction)
  - athetoid gait
  - limp (antalgic gait)
- **Signs**
  - start by talking to the child – you may notice dysarthria
  - check eye movements for nystagmus
- Next examine **gait**
  - ataxic/trunk ataxia?
  - check for heel-to-toe walking
- **Impaired coordination**
  - on finger–nose testing
  - intention tremor
  - past pointing
  - dysdiadochokinesis (testing the ability to perform rapidly alternating movements)
  - impaired coordination on heel–shin testing

Look for other clues:

- Bruising or other evidence of falls
- Signs of neurosurgical scars/shunts
- Evidence of chemotherapy or radiotherapy
- Look at the feet – Friedreich ataxia is associated with pes cavus
- State you would like to examine the vision and fundi – Friedreich ataxia may be associated with optic atrophy

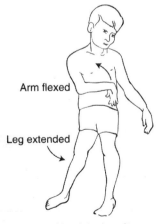
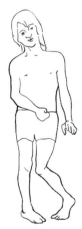
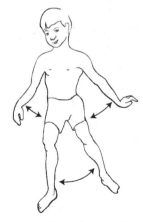

Arm flexed

Leg extended

Hemiplegic gait   Waddling gait   Broad based arms out, Ataxic gait

FIGURE 5.6 Abnormal gaits.

What is your differential diagnosis of cerebellar signs in a child?

- Neoplastic lesion/space-occupying lesion in cerebellum, e.g. neuroblastoma
- After infections, e.g. varicella causing a cerebellar encephalopathy
- Toxins, e.g. alcohol, phenytoin
- Ataxic cerebral palsy
- Spinocerebellar atrophy/Friedreich ataxia
- Ataxia telangiectasia

What other associations are there with Friedreich ataxia?

- Ataxia
- Loss of proprioception and vibration
- Loss of tendon reflexes
- Pes cavus
- Diabetes
- Optic atrophy
- Cardiomyopathy

It often presents between the ages of 8 and 15 years.

What do you know of the inheritance of Friedreich ataxia?

Autosomal recessive.

Hereditary sensory motor neuropathy (HSMN)

Also known as Charcot–Marie–Tooth/peroneal muscular atrophy.

Observation

- Callipers/foot splints/arch supports
- Gait – high-stepping gait of foot drop
- Champagne bottle legs – distal/peroneal muscle wasting
- Pes cavus – claw toes
- Claw hands/wasting of small muscles of the hands
- Evidence of neuropathic ulcers on feet/burns on hands
- Inspection of back for scoliosis

Examination

- Palpable peripheral nerves in some patients
- Tone, power, reflexes, sensation:
  - muscle weakness
  - loss of knee and ankle reflexes
  - impaired proprioception/sensation

Other associated features

Occasionally associated with retinitis pigmentosa, optic atrophy or hearing problems.

What do you know about the inheritance?

Different forms, e.g. HSMN-1 and -2. Variable inheritance – autosomal dominant, autosomal recessive and X-linked forms.

How would you diagnose the condition?

- Nerve conduction studies
- Genetic testing

How would you manage a child with HSMN?

- Genetic counselling
- Physiotherapy
- Footwear/podiatry involvement, importance of looking after feet
- Corrective foot/scoliosis surgery may be required
- Follow up by orthopaedics
- Calipers or walking aids may be required
- Consider a medic alert bracelet as in the event of an emergency, anaesthetists would need to know about the condition (www.medicalert.org.uk)
- Support groups/further information is available at, for example, www.cmt.org.uk

Common syndromes

Hypothyroidism and hyperthyroidism

Table 5.1 shows the different clinical features of hypothyroidism and hyperthyroidism.

Sturge–Weber syndrome

- Associated with epilepsy, learning disabilities and hemiplegia
- Sporadic condition
- Haemangiomatous facial lesions in the fifth cranial nerve distribution associated with haemangiomata of the meninges. This always affects the ophthalmic division and often the maxillary and mandibular divisions as well

Skull X-ray shows cerebral calcification. Differential diagnosis of cerebral calcification includes:

- Arteriovenous malformations
- Toxoplasmosis
- Cytomegalovirus
- Glioma/astrocytoma
- Craniopharyngioma

Lysosomal enzyme storage disorders

- Mucopolysaccharidoses (Hunter and Hurler syndromes)
- Lipid storage disorders: Tay–Sachs, Gaucher, Niemann–Pick

Hurler syndrome

Autosomal recessive disorder. Developmental delay from 6–12 months. Features include:

- Clouding of cornea
- Glaucoma
- Coarse facial features

- Large tongue
- Excess hair
- Bones – thick skull, kyphosis in thoracolumbar region
- Heart – valvular lesions and heart failure
- Neurodevelopment – regressive development
- Hepatosplenomegaly

Hunter syndrome

X-linked recessive disorder. No corneal clouding and less severe changes.

Chromosomal disorders

Down syndrome (trisomy 21)

This is the commonest chromosomal abnormality seen in practice. The clinical features and bio–psycho–social implications are considered more fully in Chapters 3 and 7. Down syndrome can affect several organ systems and the child commonly has characteristic dysmorphic features. Children with Down syndrome frequently participate in paediatric examinations. *Know this condition and its associated features.*

Turner syndrome (Figure 5.7)

Chromosomes: XO. Incidence 1/2000–2500.

Noonan syndrome

This is the male version of Turner syndrome but is now known to occur in both sexes. The incidence is 1/2000 and the features as follows:

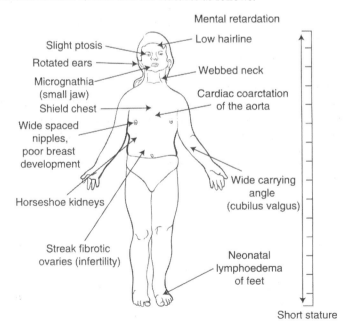

FIGURE 5.7   Features of Turner syndrome..

- Downward sloping palpebral fissures
- High-arched palate
- Webbing of neck
- Short stature
- Pectus excavatum
- Right heart abnormalities including atrial septal defect and pulmonary stenosis

Williams syndrome

- Supravalvular aortic stenosis
- Learning disabilities
- Notable feature: transient neonatal hypercalcaemia

Prader–Willi syndrome

The incidence is 1/10 000 and it is a deletion of the long arm of chromosome 15. Features include:

- Hypotonia in neonates
- Later development of obesity
- Hypogonadism
- Developmental delay
- Small hands and feet
- Short stature
- Scoliosis

Top tips

- Introduce yourself and establish a rapport with the child and parent
- Listen carefully to the examiner's instructions
- Only examine what is asked for
- Do not take a history
- Do not be put off by the examiner interrupting to ask questions
- State how you would complete your clinical assessment, particularly if only part of a system examination is asked for, and remember in paediatrics any clinical assessment must include the child's weight, height and head circumference plotted in the PCHR

Anchor statement: clinical assessment

Station 5: Clinical assessment		
	Expected standard **CLEAR PASS**	**PASS**
RAPPORT	Full greeting and introduction Clarifies role and agrees aims and objectives Good eye contact and posture Perceived to be actively listening (nod etc.) with verbal and non-verbal cues Appropriate level of confidence Empathetic nature Putting parent/child at ease	Adequately performed but not fully fluent in conducting interview
CLINICAL SKILLS	Appropriate level of confidence Well-structured and systematic examination Correctly identifies and interprets clinical signs and differential diagnosis Suggests appropriate management	Majority of clinical skills demonstrated accurately eliciting the majority of physical signs correctly Identifies majority of signs correctly May need some prompting and may be some lack of fluency

© Royal College of Paediatrics and Child Health 2012, reproduced with permission.

BARE FAIL	CLEAR FAIL	UNACCEPTABLE
Incomplete or hesitant greeting and introduction Inadequate identification of role, aims and objectives Poor eye contact and posture Not perceived to be actively listening (nod etc.) with verbal and non-verbal cues Does not show appropriate level of confidence, empathetic nature or putting parent/child at ease	Significant components omitted or not achieved	Dismissive of parent/child concerns Fails to put parent or child at ease
Too many minor errors Examination technique not well structured Non-fluent approach	Misses several important clinical signs Slow, uncertain, unstructured, unsystematic examination	Misses crucial important clinical signs or potentially dangerous interpretation Rough handling of child Disregards child's distress or shyness or modesty

6 FOCUSED HISTORY AND MANAGEMENT PLANNING

The history forms the crux of most diagnoses. Therefore, it is essential that you are skilled at taking a focused and accurate history, from which you can then formulate a management plan.

This station assesses your ability to ask pertinent questions, succinctly summarize the history, and explore management options.

Format

You will be given the scenario brief to read 2 minutes prior to the station. Upon entering the station you will be introduced to the parent and/or child from whom you will take the history and discuss management options. After 6 minutes, the parent and/or child will leave and you will have 3 minutes of discussion with the examiner. During these 3 minutes, you will be expected to succinctly summarize the history and discuss your management plan.

How to approach this station

You should aim to use the 2 minutes before entering the station to prepare your questions for the focused history. Think about jotting them down quickly and use them for reference, in case your nerves take over and you lose your chain of thought during the station.

Good communication skills form an inherent part of this assessment. Make sure you establish a good rapport with the parent and/or child by warmly introducing yourself, clarifying the objectives, demonstrating an empathic and supportive nature and encouraging their input using your non-verbal communication skills. If the child is present, then fully involve them in the history taking, aiming for a relaxed discussion with both the child and the parent.

You will need to obtain a thorough history about the current problem as well as some background history. The station is not a test of your ability to take a complete history and you are unlikely to be asked to present everything that you have just learned to the examiner. Nevertheless, remember to cover the past medical history (PMH), drug history and other relevant areas (e.g. family history (FH)). If the parent or child asks a question during the history, then you must answer it.

During this station, remember that there are two 'assessments'; one consists of the focused history and the other component is your discussion with the examiner. Marks may be given for:

- Establishing a good rapport
- Asking clear and structured questions pertinent to the case
- Appropriately answering the parent's/child's questions
- Avoiding jargon, picking up verbal and non-verbal cues
- Inviting further questions
- Succinctly summarizing the key issues
- Giving accurate information
- Exploring management options
- Providing further contact information
- Referring to other agencies when appropriate

If you are running out of time, acknowledge and explain this to the parent and/or child. Close the discussion sensibly by summarizing, offering follow up and written information.

> **Top tips**
> • Prepare wisely during the 2 minutes before the station and jot down your questions for the history taking
> • Remember to cover the past medical history, drug history and other relevant areas (e.g. family history)

Common themes

These stations often involve children with a chronic illness, so you should be familiar with the management of common childhood illnesses and chronic conditions. The topics are often chronic diseases such as:

- Diabetes
- Asthma
- Epilepsy
- Eczema
- Nocturnal enuresis
- Cystic fibrosis

Skills to demonstrate

Use the Anchor statements (pp. 116–117), reproduced with permission from the RCPCH, to understand what the examiners will be looking for. You can use it as a 'mark scheme' to grade your performance when doing the practice cases.

Worked examples

This chapter gives examples of scenarios that you could practise with a colleague. Remember that this is a clinical examination and practise is vital. The scenarios also illustrate your need to think of the child and their family as a whole when planning the management. You should include psychological aspects, the need to refer to other agencies and the availability of other sources of information for the family, as well as the medical management.

Asthma

Role: You are a GP

Setting: GP surgery

Scenario: You are talking to Peter, a 10-year-old boy, and his mother

Task: Take a focused history for this case and discuss your management plan with the examiner

Background information: A couple and their 10-year-old son, who has asthma, have just moved to your area. Peter is attending your surgery for the first time with his mother

---

You should:

1. Introduce yourself and establish a rapport. If the son is with his parents, interact with him too.
2. Explain that you need to ask them some questions about his asthma so that you can ensure that he is properly managed.
3. Start with open-ended questions:
   - How are things going with his asthma at the moment?
   - Do you have any concerns?
4. Then ask focused questions:
   Determine the severity/history of his asthma
   - How long has he had asthma?
   - How bad is it? Has hospital admission ever been necessary? Has he been admitted to an intensive care unit?
   - Has he been given any courses of steroids?
   - Has he needed time off school?
   - Does he cough and have disturbed sleep?
   - Is he coping with physical education at school/keeping up with peers/friends when playing?
   - Do you keep a peak flow diary?
   - Is he growing OK?
   Current management
   - What medication does he currently use?
   - Is he happy with his spacer/inhaler type?
   - How does he use it – washing out mouth after inhaled steroid use?
   What tends to trigger his asthma?
   - Hayfever?
   - Allergies?
   - Eczema?

- Pets?
- Smoking – parents? Smoky rooms?

5. Take a quick background history (depending on time available and what you feel is relevant)
   - PMH
   - Medication
   - Allergies
   - FH of asthma?
   - Social history (SH) – family structure
   - Immunizations
   - Development/school
   - Birth

6. Plan for care
   - Whose care is he under? (practice asthma nurse/hospital paediatric respiratory clinic?)
   - How often is he seen?
   - Do they have a plan for what to do when he gets a cough/cold?

7. Summarize what you have discussed with them.
   - Ask if they have any more questions

8. Depending on the answers you get it may be appropriate to:
   - Arrange follow up with an asthma nurse/yourself
   - Refer to a paediatrician
   - Ask them to keep a peak flow diary
   - Review or alter medication
   - Check inhaler techniques/teach about spacer
   - Offer allergen/smoking advice
   - Educate them so that they know what to do in an exacerbation (with written information)
   - Offer information, e.g. websites/support groups

A useful website with leaflets and advice for children and parents is available at www.asthma.org.uk.

Familiarize yourself with the latest asthma guidelines – particularly helpful are the British Thoracic Society (BTS)/Scottish Intercollegiate Guidelines Network (SIGN) guidelines (www.brit-thoracic.org.uk, www.sign.ac.uk). The paediatric British National Formulary (BNFc) has useful information on asthma medications and the stepwise approach that should be adopted (bnfc.org/bnfc).

Cystic fibrosis

Children with this condition are commonly encountered in the DCH and you should be able to examine and discuss in some detail the relevant clinical signs. Refresh your knowledge before the examination by reading about the clinical features and management of cystic fibrosis in a paediatric textbook.

> **Role:** You are a GP
> **Setting:** GP surgery
> **Scenario:** You are talking to Cheryl, a 13-year-old girl and her mother
> **Task:** Take a focused history for this case and discuss your management plan with the examiner
> **Background information:** Cheryl is a 13-year-old girl who is missing a lot of school due to her cystic fibrosis and she is losing weight. Mum is concerned

1. Introduce yourself to Cheryl and her mum and explain your role. Establish a rapport.
2. Start with open-ended questions:
   - [to the mother] What are your concerns?
   - [To Cheryl] How do you see the problem?
   - How much school does she miss and why? Is she falling behind? What would help her to miss less school?
   - Why do they think she is losing weight?
3. Then ask more focused questions:
   - When was she diagnosed?
   - How does it affect her now?
   - What is her current management?
   - Who is she receiving treatment from? (community specialist nurse, specialist centre, local paediatric team, community paediatrician, other specialists, e.g. gastroenterology)
   - How often is she followed up?
4. In order to determine why she might be losing weight/missing school it may be helpful to consider one system at a time:
   Respiratory
   - Is she often off school with chest infections?
   - Does she use inhalers? Antibiotics? Does she have a permanent line (e.g. portacath) for intravenous antibiotics?
   - What physiotherapy does she do? Postural drainage? Does she do any at school?
   - How many hospital admissions has she had?
   Gastroenterology
   - What dietary supplements does she take?
   - How much weight has she lost?
   - Does she take her Creon? (pancreatic enzyme supplement)
   - How is her appetite?
   - Is she opening her bowels OK? Stool – any steatorrhoea? Rectal prolapse?
   - Any abdominal pain or jaundice?
   Cardiac
   - Is she under a cardiologist?
   - Has she had an echocardiogram?
   - What is her exercise tolerance like?
   Endocrine
   - Are there any symptoms of diabetes?

- Has she been checked for diabetes?
- Where is she in relation to puberty?
- Has she had her adolescent growth spurt?

Psychological

- How is she coping with cystic fibrosis as a teenager?
- Are there any support groups in the area?
- Has she ever had any counselling?
- Does anything worry her or make her feel down?
- Does she suffer from low mood or tearfulness?
- Does she get embarrassed about taking medications/doing physiotherapy at school?

You could then summarize the key points of the case and discuss the management of her cystic fibrosis.

Ask if she or her mother have any questions.

5. Depending on the answers you get it may be appropriate to:
   - Discuss the need for further investigations into her weight loss
   - Refer her to a hospital paediatrician and a dietician
   - Treat her psychological well-being with counselling/support groups
   - Liaise with community child health teams/school – to try and address school absence (explore possibility of home-based teaching when she is unwell)

She may be interested in looking at the Cystic Fibrosis Trust website, which provides useful information/support (www.cftrust.org.uk).

Epilepsy

Read about the common types of epilepsy in young children. Remember that children who have had a single fit are not usually diagnosed immediately with epilepsy or started on medications.

Role: You are a GP

Setting: GP surgery

Scenario: You are talking to Sam, a 10-year-old boy and his mother

Task: Take a focused history for this case and discuss your management plan with the examiner

Background information: Sam is a 10-year-old with epilepsy. His mum is concerned about him going on a school trip as his epilepsy is not well controlled at present

---

1. Introduce yourself to Sam and his mum and build a rapport.

2. Explain that you understand her worries and that you will need to ask a few questions about her son's epilepsy in order to plan what to do about the school trip.

3. Start with open-ended questions:
   - What will the trip involve?
   - How will the children be supervised?
   - Are the school staff members trained in what to do if he fits? Do they carry rectal diazepam or buccal midazolam?

4. Then ask more focused questions:
   - When was he diagnosed?
   - What medication is he on?
   - Is he experiencing any side effects?
   - Is he compliant?
   - Has there been any recent change in medication?
   - Has he been followed up/by whom?
   - Does he have an alert bracelet?
   - What is his fit frequency?
   - What triggers his fits?
   - Does he experience an aura and warning signs?
   - How would he be treated if he fits?
   - How is his general development and progress at school?
   - Psychological effects – how does he feel about the epilepsy?
   - Do you have any support? Have you ever been on outings with an epilepsy support group?
   - How do his friends react?

5. Summarize what the mother has told you and what her concerns are

6. Ask if she has any more questions

7. Depending on the answers you get it may be appropriate to discuss:
   - Referral to a paediatrician for optimization of his medications
   - Mum to check the level of supervision on the trip – negotiation about which activities would and would not be safe (e.g. lone swimming or cycling)
   - Importance of compliance with medications
   - Awareness by Sam of triggers, e.g. hunger/overtiredness
   - Wearing a Medicalert bracelet
   - Liaison with school (is there a school nurse?) and education for his school regarding management of his epilepsy
   - Provision of emergency rectal diazepam/buccal midazolam (for home and school)
   - Referral to epilepsy support groups

The website www.epilepsy.org.uk has lots of information for children, adolescents and their families, and for friends who may want to learn more.

Look at the BNF to familiarize yourself with the common antiepileptic drugs and their side effects (bnfc.org/bnfc), e.g.:

- Phenytoin – gum hypertrophy, coarse facies, acne and hirsutism, tremor and ataxia

● Carbamazepine – rashes, blood disorders, drowsiness, visual disturbance
● Sodium valproate – liver toxicity, weight gain, nausea

Remember to educate teenage girls on contraception (enzyme induction makes hormonal contraception less effective and antiepileptic drugs can be teratogenic).

Diabetes

> **Role:** You are a GP
> **Setting:** GP surgery
> **Scenario:** You are talking to Brian a 14-year-old boy and his father
> **Task:** Take a focused history for this case and discuss your management plan with the examiner
> **Background information:** Brian has just moved to your area. He is a diabetic and is 14 years old. His dad has brought him in as he is concerned that his sugars are not well controlled and Brian is not really bothering to check his levels

1. Introduce yourself to Brian and his dad and establish a rapport.
2. Explain that you would like to find out a bit more about his diabetes so that you can address their concerns.
3. Start with open-ended questions:
   ● [To dad] What are your concerns about the diabetes at the moment?
   ● [To Brian] How do you feel about your diabetic control at the moment?
4. Then ask more focused questions:
   ● What treatment is he on at the moment?
   ● Does he give his own injections?
   ● Does he vary the sites of injections? Does he have any problems with injection sites?
   ● When does he check his blood sugars? How does he feel about that?
   ● What sort of readings is he getting? Does he keep a diary?
   ● Does he ever check his urine for ketones?
   ● Does he ever miss doses?
   ● Are there any hypoglycaemic attacks (hypos)? What does he do if he gets a hypo? What warning does he get? Do his family members and school know how to treat one? Does he carry a source of sugar with him, e.g. Hypostop/Lucozade tablets?
   ● Has he ever been admitted with diabetic ketoacidosis?
   ● Does he know what to do if he is ill?
   ● What is his exercise level like/is he involved in any particular sport?
   ● How is his diet?
   ● How is his weight?
   ● Where is he in relation to puberty? Has he had a recent growth spurt?
   ● How does he manage his diabetes at school?
   ● How do his friends react?
   ● Does it bother him to inject at school?

- What is his psychological state?
- Are there any known problems with: injection sites?, feet?, eyes?, kidneys?

5. Ask Brian if he has any concerns/worries
6. Summarize the main issues and concerns that have been raised
7. Ask if there are any more questions
8. Depending on the answers you get it may be appropriate to:
   - Refer to a paediatrician
   - Arrange follow up with a specialist diabetic nurse/yourself
   - Consider testing thyroid function and performing a coeliac screen (there is an increased incidence)
   - Adjust medications/monitoring so they fit better into the teenager's life
   - Work on education about hypos/what to do when unwell
   - Liaise with school – education on diabetes/management of hypos
   - Refer to dietician
   - Consider psychological support/referral to support group
   - Offer advice on where to find more information on the Internet

The website www.diabetes.org.uk includes a section entitled 'My life', which is geared to young people with diabetes; www.nice.org.uk has a quick reference guide entitled 'Type 1 diabetes in children and young people', and www.library.nhs. uk/diabetes has a very useful document called 'Approaching the parents of a child with diabetes'. The latter makes many suggestions for parents looking after a child with diabetes, e.g. they advise that rewards should be offered for sticking to the correct diet and complying with treatment. They should never depend on outcomes, e.g. HbA1C.

Enuresis

Role: You are a GP

Setting: GP surgery

Scenario: You are talking to Donald's mother

Task: Take a focused history for this case and discuss your management plan with the examiner

Background information: Donald's mum has come to see you about him as he is 7 years old and is still wetting the bed

---

1. Introduce yourself and establish a rapport.
2. Explain that you will need to ask some questions about Donald and then you will be able to decide how best to help him.
3. Start with open-ended questions:
   - Ask about the problem and her concerns
   - Why is she concerned now?
   - What does she think is causing it?
4. Then ask more focused questions:
   - What is the history of his potty training?
   - Is he dry during the day?

- Has he ever been dry at night?
- How often does he wet the bed?
- What do they do when he wets the bed? What have they tried: fluid restriction in the evening or waking him to go to the toilet when parents go to bed?
- Is anything bothering him, i.e. stress at school or home?
- Are there any symptoms of infection – tummy pains, fever or complaints of discomfort on passing urine?
- Are there any symptoms of diabetes – increased fluid intake, thirst, weight change, infections?
- Are there problems with constipation?

5. Take a quick background history (depending on time available and what you feel is relevant)
   - PMH – is there spina bifida or diabetes?
   - Medications/allergies
   - FH of enuresis – brothers/sisters/father?
   - SH – family structure? New baby? Any stress at home?
   - Immunizations
   - Development/school – is there any stress or concerns about school?
   - Birth

6. Summarize the issues/concerns raised by his mum

7. Ask if there are any more questions. Depending on the answers you get it may be appropriate to:
   - Arrange to see Donald to perform an examination
   - Talk to Donald about the problem and offer reassurance
   - Perform further investigations including testing for diabetes and urinary infection
   - Refer to a specialist
   - Offer psychological support
   - Teach family behavioural techniques such as star charts
   - Talk about fluids, e.g. drinking a reasonable amount in the day, avoiding fizzy drinks and using the toilet before bed
   - Offer more specialized equipment such as pad alarms (usually only effective in 7 years+), waterproof sheeting

Discuss short-term medications such as desmopressin for school trips etc., however drugs are used less and less frequently. Tricyclics such as imipramine are now contraindicated due to the risk of serious cardiac arrhythmias in overdose and there has been a drug safety alert for use of desmopressin following its link to concerns about water retention and seizures (www.mhra.gov.uk).

Inform them of websites/help groups and sources of further information/leaflets, e.g. from Education and Resources for Improving Childhood incontinence (ERIC) www.eric.org.uk.

Common treatment options for nocturnal enuresis include:

- Dry bed training refers to regimens that include enuresis alarms, waking routines, positive practise, cleanliness training, bladder training and rewards in various combinations.

- Star charts are used as a record and incentive scheme, alone or with other treatments.
- Enuresis alarms, which wake the child in the night at the onset of wetting, are a form of conditioning that may require several months of continual use to be effective.
- Desmopressin is a synthetic analogue of antidiuretic hormone that reduces nocturnal urine output. It has a rapid onset, making it suitable for short-term use. It can be used alone or with an enuresis alarm. The indication has been withdrawn for the nasal spray form, Desmospray, due to the risk of side effects in overdose (water intoxication/hyponatraemia)

Headache

> **Role:** You are a GP
> **Setting:** GP surgery
> **Scenario:** You are talking to Eleanor's mother
> **Task:** Take a focused history for this case and discuss your management plan with the examiner
> **Background information:** Eleanor is missing a lot of school due to headaches. Her mother is concerned

1. Introduce yourself to Eleanor and her mum and build a rapport
2. Start with open-ended questions:
   - Can you tell me about the headaches?
   - What do you think is causing them?
   - What are you worried about?
   - How much school is she missing?
   - Is she falling behind?
3. Then ask more focused questions:
   - How long have the headaches been going on for? When did they first start?
   - Are there any warning/triggers?
   - Onset?
   - Location?
   - Character?
   - How long do they last for?
   - Is there any pattern to the headaches? (time of day/day of week? Worse first thing in the morning, better at weekends?)
   - Have they become progressively worse? Is the pattern changing?
   - How does she look when she has the headache?
   - Are there any associated symptoms: vomiting, nausea, fever, photophobia, weight loss?
   - How do they treat the headaches? What helps? What makes them worse?
   Are there any other problems or symptoms?
   - Is she growing well/progressing at school OK?

- Is her eyesight OK?
- Is she clumsy, and is her reading/writing deteriorating?
- Is she enjoying school/a recent change in school?
- Is there anything she does not like at school?
- Is there any bullying going on?

4. Take a quick background history (depending on time available and what you feel is relevant)
   - PMH – are there any other illnesses?
   - Medications/allergies – is there an overuse of analgesics? (analgesic or rebound headache)
   - Is there a FH of migraines?
   - Is there a SH – family structure? Is there any stress at home? Depression? Bereavement?
   - What is her history of immunizations?
   - Development/school – is there any stress or concerns about school?
   - What was her birth like?

5. Summarize the issues/concerns raised by the patient's mother

6. Ask if there are any more questions. Depending on the answers you get it may be appropriate to:
   - Arrange to examine Eleanor (check blood pressure, growth, neurological examination including fundi, dermatological examination for neurocutaneous lesions)
   - Arrange an eye test
   - Ask her and her mother to keep a diary of her symptoms
   - Offer reassurance
   - Explain that a scan is not necessary (unless there are red flags such as an abnormal neurological examination, seizures, a recent onset of severe headache, early morning headaches, vomiting, deterioration in writing/school performance)
   - Talk about migraines running in the family
   - Talk about treatment
   - Refer to a paediatrician
   - Liaise with the school
   - Explore psychological issues
   - Offer leaflets/sources of more information
   - Offer a follow-up appointment

The UCL Institute of Child Health has produced some useful paediatric guidelines including one on 'headache' (www.ich.ucl.ac.uk).

Crying baby

> **Role:** You are a GP
>
> **Setting:** GP surgery
>
> **Scenario:** You are talking to Mrs Smith
>
> **Task:** Take a focused history for this case and discuss your management plan with the examiner
>
> **Background information:** Mrs Smith is concerned that her 2-month-old baby has been crying a lot over the last few weeks and she doesn't know what is wrong

1. Introduce yourself to the mother and build a rapport
2. Start with some open-ended questions:
   - Can you tell me about your new baby?
   - What do you think is causing the crying?
   - What are you worried about?
   - What does your health visitor/family think?
3. Then ask more focused questions:
   - When does the crying occur?
   - What time of day/night does it occur?
   - Is there a relationship to feeds?
   - Are there periods of contentment?
   - What does the baby look like – flushed/pale/legs drawn up?
   - What do you do when the baby cries?
   - What seems to help?
   - Feeding pattern – breast/bottle?
   - How much milk? When?
   - Is the baby gaining weight? Is the head circumference OK?
   - Have you brought the Personal Child Health Record (PCHR, red book) with her?
   - What are the stools like?
   - Is she producing wet nappies?
   - Is there any vomiting?
   - Is there any nappy rash or skin rashes?
   - Is there any fever?
   - Are there any other symptoms?
4. Take a quick background history (depending on time available and what you feel is relevant)
   - Medications/allergies – what have you tried giving?
   - FH – do you have any other children? Did they have similar problems when they were young?
   - SH – family structure? Is there any stress at home? Are there any other children at home?
   - Do you have any family support? Parents? Is your husband/partner at home?

5. Take a birth history
   - Were there any problems in the neonatal period?
   - Did the baby pass meconium in the first 24 hours?
   - Did the baby spend time in the special care baby unit?
   - Was the baby born prematurely?
6. Do a psychological assessment
   - Are there signs of postnatal depression?
   - Is she coping with the tiredness?
   - Does she get any help at night?
   - Is the stress affecting her relationship with her husband/partner?
   - What support does she have?
7. Summarize the problem and the mother's concerns
8. Ask if there are any more questions. Depending on the answers you get it may be appropriate to:
   - Arrange to examine the baby to look for causes, e.g. nappy rash, oral thrush
   - Check head circumference/weight and plot in PCHR (red book)
   - Arrange further investigations
   - Refer to a paediatrician
   - Offer reassurance if this is a well baby who has periods of contentment and is gaining weight well
   - Discuss remedies such as Infacol (simeticone) if the pattern of crying is mostly in the evenings and suggestive of colic; some mothers find it helps
   - Is the baby overfed, prematurely weaned or inadvertently swallowing air at the end of a bottle feed? Advice on feeding may be needed
   - Involve a health visitor
   - Arrange support for the mother – encourage parents to get as much rest as possible, perhaps asking a family member to babysit for a period
   - Screen mum for postnatal depression
   - Give advice on parenting groups for support
   - Offer a follow-up visit
   - Offer sources of further information, e.g. the Internet

Birth to Five (www.dh.gov.uk) is a very useful source of sensible advice on feeding, immunizations, childhood illnesses, child safety, child development, practical support and benefits for parents. The DCH covers common childhood problems and this source explains things in simple language that can help you explain various issues to parents in the communication as well as history stations. You could also suggest the book to a parent who wanted more information.

Practice cases

Note: there is an overlap between topics that can appear in these stations and those that test communications skills:

- Child with a disability moving to your area
- Child with trisomy 21 (Down syndrome)
- Poor eating/picky eater/obesity
- Behavioural problems such as tantrums, not sleeping, hyperactivity, autistic spectrum disorder
- Chronic abdominal pain
- Review of eczema
- Constipation
- Failure to thrive

Anchor statement: focused history and management planning

Station 6: Focused history		
	Expected standard **CLEAR PASS**	**PASS**
PART A: RAPPORT	Full greeting and introduction Clarifies role and agrees aims and objectives Good eye contact and posture Perceived to be actively listening (nod etc.) with verbal and non- verbal cues Appropriate level of confidence Empathetic nature Putting parent/child at ease	Adequately performed but not fully fluent in conducting interview
PART A: **FOCUSED HISTORY**	Ask clear question pertinent to the case Use open and closed questions. Parent, child and examiner can hear and understand fully Appropriate answers to parents' questions Structured questions, avoids jargon, picks up verbal and non- verbal cues Succinct summary of key issues	Questions reasonable and cover essential issues but omits occasional essential points Overall approach structured Appropriate style of questioning Main points summarized
PART B: SUMMARY, **MANAGEMENT** **PLANNING AND** **CLOSURE**	Invites further questions Summarizes Gives accurate information Explores options for management Provides appropriate further contact	Summarizes most of the important points and suggests best management strategy Provides some information about other services and future plan

© Royal College of Paediatrics and Child Health 2012, reproduced with permission.

BARE FAIL	CLEAR FAIL	UNACCEPTABLE
Incomplete or hesitant greeting and introduction Inadequate identification of role, aims and objectives Poor eye contact and posture Not perceived to be actively listening (nod etc.) with verbal and non-verbal cues Does not show appropriate level of confidence, empathetic nature or putting parent/child at ease	Significant components omitted or not achieved	Dismissive of parent/child concerns Fails to put parent or child at ease
Misses relevant information, that would make a difference to management if known Excessive use of closed question Occasional use of jargon Summary incomplete	Asks irrelevant questions, poorly understood by parent and child Excessive use of jargon Does not seek the view of parent/child Very poor summary	Questions totally unrelated to the problem presented. Shows no regard to the child/parent No summary
Incomplete summary of problems and inadequately planned management Does not relate management to child/parents needs or concerns Inadequate attempt to determine child/parent understanding	Poor summary Patient unsure of future plans Poor discussion of management options	Abrupt ending Inaccurate information given Lack of regard for safe, ethical and effective treatments

7

CHILD DEVELOPMENT

As a GP, you are expected to have a sound knowledge of the developmental milestones and be able to detect abnormalities, whilst reassuring parents that their child is within the normal range.

This station is designed to test your ability to perform a clinical developmental assessment, and to discuss the implications of your findings and potential management. You may also be asked to comment on neurodisability or use supplementary information such as a growth chart or brief history from the parent if appropriate.

Format

You will be given the brief once you have entered the station and the examiner will introduce you to the child and parent/carer. Remember this station comprises two assessments, so you will have 6 minutes to perform your developmental assessment, and 3 minutes for discussion with the examiner.

It can be difficult to perform a comprehensive developmental assessment within this short time, but by using a systematic approach you should be able to make a good estimate of the child's age, or if this has been given to you, assess whether the child's development is normal. The examiners will offer direction if appropriate.

How to approach this station

The key things to remember for any developmental assessment are the following four main areas. Break down your assessment and ensure that you touch on all of these four areas in your examination:

1. Gross motor
2. Fine motor and vision
3. Hearing and communication
4. Socialization

Usually, this station will focus on one area in particular, so listen carefully to the instructions. Even if the abnormality appears to be in one area only, you will need to quickly check other areas to ensure that the child does not have a global developmental delay. Therefore, for a complete developmental assessment, you should always consider the other areas, ask to see the red book (Personal Child Health Record – PCHR) and offer to measure weight, head circumference and height and plot these on a growth chart.

There is no rigid structure to assessing development, but you should have a systematic approach to make sure you cover all the key components. Nevertheless, be flexible and do not allow the child to get bored. Keep introducing new toys or things to do, and praise the child at each step. You should smile, be encouraging and make the tasks into a game where possible. Remember that your rapport, interaction, body language and communication skills will also be assessed during your time at this station.

During this assessment you should aim to elicit and demonstrate to the examiner the key developmental milestones via your examination. Sometimes it may be necessary to ask the parent a couple of questions whilst observing the child during your examination, however you should check that this is the case with the examiner prior to asking the parent any questions.

There will be numerous toys, books and aids in the room for you to select. The onus is on you to set up an age-appropriate situation in order to assess the child's development. Take a moment to step back and observe the child playing in the environment initially. Then you should become involved by getting down to the child's level and joining them in their play. By using the apparatus available as aids, you should be able gently to guide the child to illustrate key milestones.

In this station, the child's developmental age will be less than 4 years. You must learn and be able to apply the developmental milestones up to this age at least. Familiarity with the milestones will make it easy for you to find things that a child can do, then something that they cannot and thereby narrow down their likely age. Remember, there is no substitute for practise. It will be obvious to the examiner if you have not practised these skills.

During your discussion with the examiner, you should succinctly summarize your findings and include relevant information elicited. You should demonstrate knowledge of any child development problems noted, their impact and give an appropriate management plan.

You will be assessed on your general approach and whether it is systematic. You should communicate clearly what you wish a child to do, and be able to identify normal and abnormal development. Your ability to explain or summarize the findings and decide on a sensible management plan such as investigations or referral will be assessed.

Top tips

- Start practising early
- Attend as many general and community paediatric clinics as possible
- Listen carefully to the instructions
- Be systematic
- Practise, practise, practise!

Common themes

In this station, the child's developmental age will be less than 4 years, so make sure you know the key developmental milestones (Table 7.1) and 'red flag' signs of developmental delay.

Table 7.1 **Gross motor milestones**

Milestone	Average age achieved
Pushing up on arms when prone	3 months
Reaching for objects – bringing them to midline	3 months (should not show hand preference)
Rolling – front to back and back to front	4–6 months
Sitting	6–8 months
Crawling	9 months (look for unusual variants such as bottom shuffling that may lead to later walking)
Pulling to stand	9 months
Cruising	12 months
Walking	15 months
Can stoop and pick up ball	18 months
Kicking/throw ball	18 months
Stairs	2 years
Ride a tricycle	3 years
Jumping/hopping	4 years

Think about the approach you would take in the following station scenarios:

- 'Please assess this baby/toddler/young child's development.'
- 'This boy's parents are concerned about his vision – please assess him.'
- 'This girl's teachers are concerned about her speech – please assess her.'
- 'Please examine this baby – his mother is concerned about his hearing.'
- 'Please examine this child – she is not walking at 18 months.'

Skills to demonstrate

Use the Anchor statements (pp. 134–135), reproduced with permission from the RCPCH, to understand what the examiner will be looking for. You can use it as a 'mark scheme' to grade your performance when doing the practice cases.

Worked examples and practice cases

This chapter does not aim to provide comprehensive teaching about each aspect of child development. Instead it provides an overview and basic framework for the exam. You will find detailed tables of developmental milestones and red flags in most paediatric textbooks.

The examples below cover the essential areas that you should know for the exam. You should use the outlines given below to practise your developmental assessment and to hone your skills.

Developmental assessment

Remember to be systematic during your assessment. Take a moment to observe and inspect for any clues such as dysmorphic facies, squints, hearing aids, walking aids or specific shoes.

Gross motor assessment

- Tone – check head lag, check for spasticity
- Sit – can the child sit unsupported?
- Crawl or crawl variant
- Stand – also observe sit-to-stand ability
- Gait
- Actions – stoop, kick, throw, stairs, tricycle, jump, hop

How might a child with delayed motor development present?

A child with delayed motor development often presents as a floppy infant with head lag who is unable to sit unsupported. The child may show early hand preference and scissoring of the legs when lifted.

They may not be walking at 18 months and may have had crawling variants such as bottom shuffling. Note: Not all bottom shufflers go on to have problems with their motor development. Bottom shufflers may, however, be late walkers (they may not walk until age 18–24 months). This may run in families. There may be no other abnormalities but because of the link with cerebral palsy a careful examination should be carried out.

What may be the cause of developmental delay?

- Neurological problems such as cerebral palsy
- Spinal disorders such as spina bifida or spinal muscular atrophy
- Muscular disorders such as muscular dystrophy
- Myopathies such as myotonic dystrophy
- Chromosome disorders such as trisomy 21, which is associated with hypotonia
- Orthopaedic disorders such as dislocated hips or limb problems, e.g. arthrogryposis multiplex
- As part of a global developmental delay

Possible physical factors in global developmental delay include:

- Chromosome abnormality, e.g. trisomy 21
- Congenital infection
- Neonatal cerebral insult such as trauma, hypoxia, severe infection
- Use of drugs, alcohol, or teratogenic medication in pregnancy
- Physical health and nutrition of the child
- Metabolic defects
- Brain malformation

Possible psychological/social factors in developmental delay include:

- Abuse
- Neglect
- Postnatal depression
- Large family/busy mother – a child left sitting in a chair or cot all day will not be able to explore their surroundings and advance their motor skills, e.g. learning to walk

- A child who has no adult interaction may show language delay
- Cultural differences

Fine motor

- Palmar grasp – 4–6 months
- Pincer grip – scatter some hundreds and thousands or offer a small raisin – 9 months
- Draw – ask the child to draw (Table 7.2)
- Bricks – ask the child to build a tower (Table 7.3)

Table 7.2 Drawing (fine motor) milestones

Milestone	Average age
Scribble	15 months
Line	2 years
Circle	3 years
Cross	3 years
Square	4 years
Person – stick figure	4 years
Triangle	5 years

Table 7.3 Tower building with bricks (fine motor) milestones

Milestone	Average age
3 bricks	18 months
6 bricks	2 years
9 bricks	3 years

Hearing

Testing hearing depends on age:

- At birth – neonatal testing is usually carried out by otoacoustic emission testing or brainstem-evoked potentials
- Auditory brainstem response – measures electroencephalogram (EEG) waves produced in response to clicks from an electrode on the baby's scalp
- Evoked otoacoustic emissions – uses a microphone to detect sound waves emitted from hair cells in the cochlea

You should aim to visit the audiology clinic to see these tests being conducted. The red book (PCHR) contains screening questions for parents, i.e. 'Can your child hear?' Information can also be obtained from the NHS Newborn Hearing Screening Programme website (http://hearing.screening. nhs.uk/surveillance).

Distraction testing – best at around 9 months

For babies who are now screened at birth, this is no longer a routine test (Figure 7.1). However, you may be asked to demonstrate the principles of it or describe it for the examination:

- Sound proof room
- One relative only
- No distractions
- Child sitting far forward on mother's knee
- Assistant distracts the child, e.g. by moving coloured balls in her hands
- Assistant is then still and quiet, and a noise such as from a rattle (e.g. a Manchester rattle) is made just out of the child's vision at a set distance from either the right or left ear (one metre)
- Watch for a reaction from the child (turning to look for the source of the noise)
- A meter will enable frequencies and volumes to be varied and recorded

McCormack toy testing – age range 2.5–4 years (speech discrimination)

Understand the principles and if possible observe in the audiology clinic:

- There are specially made up sets of similar sounding words, e.g. horse/fork, key/tree
- First the examiner checks that the child knows what each object is
- Then, whilst covering their mouth so that the child cannot lip read, the examiner asks the child to identify various objects, e.g. 'show me the horse'

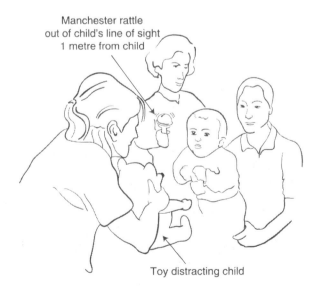

Manchester rattle
out of child's line of sight
1 metre from child

Toy distracting child

FIGURE 7.1   Distraction test. Nowadays rattle is often replaced by an electronic 'warbler'.

- Child then points to the correct object
- Examiner adjusts the volume of their voice and an assistant can use a decibel meter to record the volume
- Examiner should not use any visual clues, e.g. looking at the object they want the child to point to
- Children should get at least 8/10 correct

Younger children can perform a similar test with familiar objects, e.g. 'where is mummy?', 'where is teddy?', 'give the cup to teddy', after first checking their understanding of the object names (18–30 months).

Threshold audiometry (performance/conditioning test) – age range 21–31 months

Listening for sounds of varying intensity/frequency – younger children can be encouraged to put bricks in a box or men in a boat when they hear a noise (either pure tone audiometry, warble or voice commands), turning the test into a game and keeping the child interested. The levels are checked with a sound meter.

Initially demonstrate the exercise to the child, then help the child to carry out the task, then gradually reduce assistance until there are no visual cues and the child is carrying out the exercise alone. The child should be praised every time they correctly perform the task.

Bone conduction can be compared to air conduction if a special headset is used.

Impedence testing (tympanometry)

This uses a small piece of equipment that fits in the child's ear. It is useful for testing for glue ear (chronic secretory otitis media), which gives a flat curve.

Ensure that you can confidently perform an ear examination (Figure 7.2).

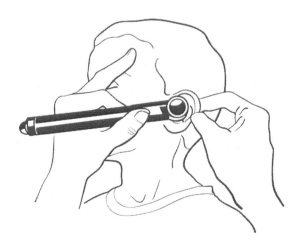

FIGURE 7.2 Examination of the ear with an auroscope.

Support and information for parents can be obtained from National Deaf Children's Society at www.ndcs.org.uk. Many aids can be provided to help a deaf child, including listening and alerting devices, subtitles, sign language tuition, communication technology, radio aids, hearing dogs, hearing aids, cochlear implants and benefits.

Risk factors for hearing loss include:

- Otitis media with effusion
- Chronic secretory otitis media
- Recurrent infections
- Drugs, e.g. gentamicin used on special care baby unit (SCBU)
- Congenital — infections, e.g. cytomegalovirus (CMV)
- Hereditary — positive family history, Down syndrome
- Prematurity
- Congenital abnormalities of head and neck development
- Kernicterus
- Meningitis — especially pneumococcal
- Developmental delay

Vision

Take parental concerns about visual impairment very seriously. Remember that severe visual impairment will impact on other aspects of development, and may be associated with underlying disorders such as Down syndrome or cerebral palsy.

Visual loss may be hereditary and progressive, such as retinitis pigmentosa. Families may need to be referred for genetic counselling.

Be aware when testing vision that the room should be well illuminated. The child's age and reading ability will determine which tests can be used (see later). Think about distance, near and colour vision.

Inspection for signs of visual problems

- Obvious abnormalities surrounding the eye, e.g. large strawberry naevus, ptosis
- Iris abnormalities, e.g. coloboma (defect in iris)
- Manifest squint (obvious)
- Visual inattention
- Random eye movements
- Nystagmus
- Photophobia
- Loss of red reflex (leucocoria)
- Not smiling responsively

Acuity assessment

If the child is wearing glasses, leave them on in order to test their corrected visual acuity. From the following ages, you should expect:

- Newborn – fixes and follows. Prefers patterned objects
- 6 months – reaches well for toys

- 9 months – picks up hundreds and thousands (tiny sweets used as cake decorations)/equivalently small items
- 2 years – matches picture cards. If testing a child who cannot yet read letters, you should show pictures of reducing size from a distance and ask the child to point to a similar picture on a card in front of them
- 3 years –matches letters using single letter charts (Sheridan and Gardner)
- 5 years –reads a Snellen chart

Squints

- Look at the position of the light on both corneas (check for the light reflex). It should fall in the same place centrally in both eyes
- Cover test – if there is a manifest/obvious squint, cover the eye that is fixing on the object. The deviated eye should move to take up fixation
- Cover–uncover test. If there is a latent squint, when you cover up one eye it stops focusing on the object and may drift out. When the eye is uncovered again, it will be seen to move back to take up fixation

There are two types of squint:
1. Concomitant (non-paralytic) (Figure 7.3):
       – convergent (esotropia)
       – divergent (exotropia)
       – alternating

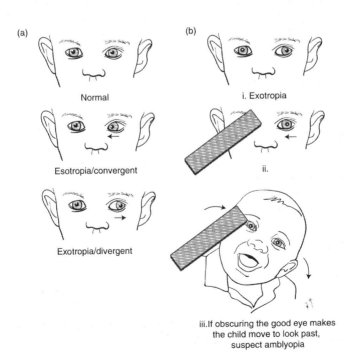

(a)

Normal

Esotropia/convergent

Exotropia/divergent

(b)

i. Exotropia

ii.

iii. If obscuring the good eye makes the child move to look past, suspect amblyopia

FIGURE 7.3   (a) Types of concomitant squint. (b) Cover test.

2. Incomitant (paralytic) – cranial nerve palsies

Pseudosquint due to prominent epicanthic folds is a fairly common finding in young babies, but if any doubt exists always refer to an orthoptist or ophthalmologist.

Colour vision assessment

Have a look at a set of Ishihara plates and learn how to interpret the results. The test consists of up to 36 cards. The patient is asked to read the hidden numbers on the cards. Eight or more errors indicate that there is a problem with colour vision.

Visual fields

In the older child, visual fields can be assessed with confrontation, as you would for an adult.

Loss of red reflex

Red reflex is the 'red eye' that may be seen in old family photographs. It would ordinarily be checked by looking at the pupils through an ophthalmoscope. The absence of red reflex requires urgent referral (see Figure 7.4).

The causes of and risk factors for visual impairment are:

- Causes:
  - retinoblastoma
  - cataract
  - retinopathy of prematurity
  - inflammatory/infectious conditions
  - chromosome disorders

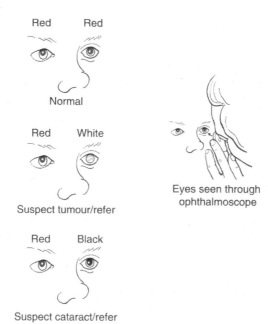

FIGURE 7.4   Red reflex abnormalities.

- squint leading to amblyopia
- amblyopia from obstructed vision, e.g. large strawberry naevus
- Risk factors:
  - prematurity
  - cerebral palsy
  - chromosome disorders such as Down syndrome
  - genetic/family history
  - congenital infection

Support and information for parents can be obtained from the National Blind Children's Society at www.nbcs.org.uk.

Speech

Listen to the child's speech. If the child is older, perhaps pick up a picture book and ask them to point to things (comprehension), ask them what the objects in the picture are and ask them to describe what is happening in the story. Children older than 2 years should be able to tell simple stories from pictures (Table 7.4). For younger children, engage them in play and ask them to play with particular toys to test their comprehension.

Table 7.4 Language milestones

Milestone	Average age
Consonant babble – baba, dada,	6 months
Using words with meaning, e.g. mama	9 months
Few words	12 months
50 words	18 months
Phrases	2 years
Sentences	3 years
Ask if they know their name	3 years
Recognizes colours	3 years
Names colours	4 years
Can count	4 years

Comment on their understanding (comprehension), expression (e.g. single words/joined words/sentences) and articulation.

Common problems that may need referral to a speech therapist include specific problems with articulation, stammers and speech delay. Remember to look for an underlying cause:

- Hearing loss
- Social factors, e.g. bullying/abuse/neglect
- Physical reason – head and neck abnormalities, cleft lip or palate, macroglossia
- Global delay
- Family history

Socialization

You may be able to observe some behaviour (Table 7.5) but also ask the examiner if you may ask the mother a few questions. Use play to elicit some of the features, such as symbolic play, for example observe if the child is pretending to cook/feed teddy some food/brush the doll's hair. If not, ask the mother about the child's play.

Table 7.5 Language milestones

Milestone	Average age
Smile	6 weeks
Wave bye-bye	9 months
Indicates wants	9 months
Clap hands	9 months
Hold cup	12 months
Feed themselves with fingers, e.g. rusk	6 months
Use spoon	15 months
Continence – dry by day	2 years
Dry by day and night	3 years
Dresses with help	3 years

Key referral criteria

You must know the age limits for referral. Table 7.6 clearly outlines the age limits for the key developmental milestones.

Table 7.6 Age limits for key developmental milestones

Milestone	Average age
Not smiling	8 weeks
Not reaching	5–6 months
Not babbling	7 months
Not sitting unassisted	9 months
No pincer grip	10–12 months
Not standing	12 months
Not saying six words	18 months
Not walking	18 months (some variants of crawling may be associated with later walking)

Note: in very premature babies you may need to allow for their prematurity in the timing of their milestones.

6-week baby check

GPs conduct the 6-week baby check. You should learn and practise this examination. Your overall inspection should determine whether the baby is well and alert. Look for signs of jaundice, dehydration or any obvious physical abnormalities:

- Fontanelle – check the anterior and posterior fontanelle (closed at term) and that they are not sunken (a sign of dehydration) or bulging (indicating raised intracranial pressure)
- Eyes – red reflex, fixing and following, squint
- Ears- any obvious abnormalities
- Facies – symmetry, low-set ears, epicanthic folds, protuberant tongue, hair line
- Palate – inspect, ask the mother about feeding difficulties and feel gently with a clean finger
- Chest – auscultate/inspect
- Arms and hands – look for any obvious problems such as polydactyly, syndactyly, single palmar crease, incurving little finger
- Abdomen – palpation, distension, masses, hernia, scars
- Umbilicus – check it is clean and dry. Check for umbilical granuloma, umbilical hernia
- Heart sounds – check for any murmurs
- Femoral pulses – check both are equal
- Hips – Barlow's and Ortolani's tests check for dislocated or dislocatable/clicky hips (Figure 7.5)
- Genitalia – look for ambiguous genitalia (this is important as it can be associated with congenital adrenal hyperplasia and a life-threatening salt-losing crisis), hypospadias (it is important to detect as parents should not have their child circumcised as there may be a need to use the foreskin for corrective surgery)
- Testis – check both are descended. If not, follow up and if persistently undescended then the baby will need to be referred for surgery (which is usually carried out before the age of 1 year old)
- Anus – patency, ask about passage of meconium. Delayed passage after birth for example may be associated with cystic fibrosis
- Legs and feet – look for equal leg length and symmetrical hip creases, talipes, femoral torsion, polydactyly. If the talipes is fixed, then refer. If it is positional, you can refer to a physiotherapist, who can show the parents some stretching exercises

(a)   (b)

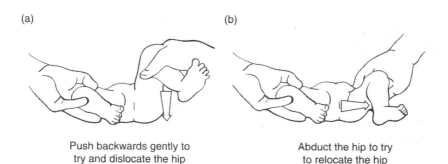

Push backwards gently to
try and dislocate the hip

Abduct the hip to try
to relocate the hip

FIGURE 7.5 (a) Barlow and (b) Ortolani tests.

- Sacrum – look for any pits/moles, which may indicate spina bifida
- Skin – note any birthmarks, e.g. strawberry naevus (Figure 7.6) (these usually regress and should be left alone unless obstructing vision or breathing/ interfering with feeding), port wine stain (cavernous haemangioma) – these usually do not fade and may need cosmetic laser treatment. If found in trigeminal nerve distribution, they may be associated with Sturge–Weber syndrome whereby there are associated intracranial abnormalities with epilepsy and intellectual impairment (Figure 7.6)
- Spine – run finger down spine, holding the baby in ventral suspension
- Head control
- Stepping reflex – hold baby upright and gently place feet on a firm surface. The baby should lift their feet in a stepping motion. Alternatively, brush the baby's shins/dorsum of feet against the side of the couch and they should make a stepping motion
- Grasp reflex – stroke the baby's palm and they will grip your finger
- Moro – support the baby in the supine position, with one hand under the head. Quickly lower the baby's head just a fraction and you will notice a flinging motion of both arms – the startle reflex. This shows that both arms are moving symmetrically, and if not, this may pick up lesions such as a brachial plexus injury sustained at birth
- Head circumference and weight (offer to plot this in the red book (PCHR)).

Questions

- Ask about family history of hip problems, heart problems or hearing/vision problems, including squint.

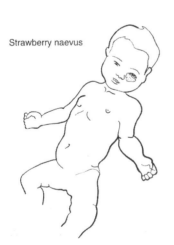
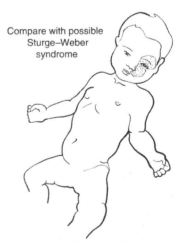

Strawberry naevus

Compare with possible Sturge–Weber syndrome

FIGURE 7.6 (a) Strawberry naevus. May present as a large pink lesion on the face as shown (or hidden behind the hairline or on the body). (b) Sturge–Weber lesion. Candidates who have not seen this before may potentially confuse this with strawberry naevus, but it is more extensive and occurs in the distribution of the trigeminal nerve.

- Check that the child has received vitamin K (oral or intramuscular (IM)), be able to discuss routes and timing of administration and the surrounding controversy).
- Discuss immunizations.
- Check that no problems were picked up on antenatal scans.
- Check that no problems were detected at neonatal hearing test.
- Ask the mother if she has any concerns.
- Watch for signs of postnatal depression, e.g. Edinburgh Postnatal Depression Score (a calculator for this can be found on www.patient.co.uk).

Common schedules of child health surveillance

As well as being familiar with the basic newborn and 6-week checks, you should be aware of other screening tests that are carried out, such as neonatal hearing testing, the heel-prick test and measurement of weight and head circumference by midwives/health visitors. GPs no longer carry out formal developmental checks after the 6-week check.

Familiarize yourself with the red book (PCHR). This keeps a record of developmental checks, weights, head circumferences and provides parents with information and advice. It can give you useful information about the types of questions that are used to flag up problems, e.g. 'Can your baby see?' or 'Can your baby hear?'

Community and specialist services

You should know the services available in your area to help children identified with any disability. These may include:

- Community/hospital paediatricians/paediatric surgeons
- Health visitors
- Specialist nurses
- Paediatric audiologists/ear, nose, throat (ENT)
- Paediatric orthoptists/ophthalmology
- Social workers
- Educational psychologists
- Statementing – special schools or support
- Physiotherapists
- Occupational therapists
- Speech and language therapists
- Dietician
- Support groups
- Respite care
- Financial support – benefits, allowances
- Specific services and education/support/equipment for those with visual or auditory problems

Anchor statement: child development

Station 7: Child development		
	Expected standard **CLEAR PASS**	**PASS**
PART A: RAPPORT	Full greeting and introduction Clarifies role and agrees aims and objectives Good eye contact and posture Perceived to be actively listening (nod etc.) with verbal and non-verbal cues Appropriate level of confidence Empathetic nature Putting parent/child at ease	Adequately performed but not fully fluent in conducting interview
PART A: **EXAMINATION OF** **CHILD**	Well structured and systematic approach Clear instructions given to child Accurate identification of normal/abnormal development and any disability	Reasonably systematic approach Identifies features of normal development
PART B: DISCUSSION OF **PROBLEMS OF CHILD** **DEVELOPMENT**	Good summary of findings and key priorities Covers relevant aspects of case, including parental views Delivers appropriate explanation Evidence of knowledge in a clinical setting Suggests appropriate investigations and referral	Adequate though not complete summary of findings and key priorities Covers main relevant aspects of case and delivers adequate explanation Appropriate investigations and referral

© Royal College of Paediatrics and Child Health 2012, reproduced with permission.

BARE FAIL	CLEAR FAIL	UNACCEPTABLE
Incomplete or hesitant greeting and introduction Inadequate identification of role, aims and objectives Poor eye contact and posture Not perceived to be actively listening (nod etc.) with verbal and non-verbal cues Does not show appropriate level of confidence, empathetic nature or putting parent/child at ease	Significant components omitted or not achieved	Dismissive of parent/child concerns Fails to put parent or child at ease
Hesitant examination covering main points but leaves out important tasks	Poorly organized, inappropriate developmental examination Poor organization of child Unable to recognize relevance of normal/abnormal signs	Completely unstructured assessment with slow hesitant approach Failure to demonstrate to child Serious inadequacy in developmental skills
Incorrect conclusion Some identification of further investigation, referral or treatment, but evidence of muddled thinking	Incorrect explanation Little clinical knowledge Poor identification of possible problems Lack of clarity of future planning	Unable to interpret findings Serious deficiencies in knowledge and understanding of child development assessment

SAFE PRESCRIBING

Safe prescribing is vital in both adult and paediatric medicine, however in paediatrics, prescribing requires greater attention because dose calculations can be complicated and small errors can cause significant harm.

This station assesses your ability to write a prescription for a child. You must prescribe correctly for the specific clinical scenario and have the correct dosage, based on the child's age and weight. You must also be able to discuss with the examiner the implications of your decisions and prescription.

Format

You will be given the scenario brief to read 2 minutes prior to starting at the station.

Upon entering the station you will have a maximum of 5 minutes to write the prescription on an FP10 (prescription form for use in community pharmacy). Then the examiner will have 4 minutes to ask you questions about your decisions and the prescription – in particular the indication, dose calculation, any contraindications or adverse reactions and specific issues relating to the medication.

Remember, this station consists of two assessments. The examiner will award a mark for your completed FP10 prescription, and then award a mark for your discussion.

How to approach this station

The basics will earn you valuable marks in this station, so don't forget to write legibly, write the child's personal details (i.e. name, address, date of birth) and complete the prescription by putting your signature, name and the date. Also remember to clearly state the route, dose, quantity per day and duration of treatment.

You will also be assessed on how confidently you select the appropriate drug and how fluently you can use the British National Formulary for Children (BNFc). For example, some candidates 'browse' through the BNFc, searching for the correct answer or information, whereas a well-prepared candidate may turn confidently to the appropriate pages and directly to the information they require. Therefore, it is important that you familiarize yourself with the BNFc.

During the discussion with the examiner, you will be required to explain your choice of medication. Your choices are likely to be based on clinical indication, national guidelines, BNFc advice and cost effectiveness. You are also likely to be asked about important side effects and contraindications of your prescribed drug. You are not expected to know all of this information verbatim, however you must have a working knowledge, access the information and be able to prescribe safely.

Key themes

The treatments for common medical conditions are likely to be tested, for example:

- Inhalers or oral medications for asthma
- Antibiotics for infections
- Antiepileptic medications
- Analgesia
- Fluids
- Insulin

The examiner may discuss the following areas:

- Dose and calculations
- Contraindications
- Adverse reactions
- Compliance issues
- Medication regimens
- Drug interactions

Skills to demonstrate

Use the Anchor statements (pp. 142–143), reproduced with permission from the RCPCH, to understand what the examiner will be looking for. You can use it as a 'mark scheme' to grade your performance when doing the practice cases.

Worked examples

> **Role:** You are a GP
> **Setting:** GP surgery
> **Scenario:** Rosie is 3 years old. She has otitis media. Prescribe a suitable antibiotic for her. Her weight is 19 kg and her height 95 cm

Amoxicillin, oral. *Note*: Amoxicillin may vary according to local protocol.

40 mg/kg daily in three divided doses (maximum 1.5 g daily in three divided doses)

Therefore, $\dfrac{40 \text{ mg/kg} \times 19 \text{ kg}}{3} = \dfrac{760}{3} = 250 \text{ mg three times a day}^{*}$

*rounded to the nearest practical dose

Amoxicillin comes as a 250 mg/5 ml suspension. Using the calculation above, this would be one 5 ml spoonful three times a day for 7 days.

Common side effects include diarrhoea, nausea and vomiting. If a rash occurs treatment should be discontinued.

If the patient is penicillin allergic or hypersensitive, then amoxicillin is contraindicated. A suitable alternative antibiotic in this case is erythromycin.

> **Role:** You are a GP
> **Setting:** GP surgery
> **Scenario:** Oscar is 7 years old. He has asthma and already uses a salbutamol inhaler as and when required. Recently mum has noticed that he coughs each night and requires the salbutamol inhaler at least five times during the week. Mum is keen for better control of his asthma. Prescribe a suitable medication for Oscar. His weight is 25 kg and height 120 cm

Based on the British Thoracic Society (BTS) guidelines, Oscar should progress to step 2 of the asthma treatment pathway – an inhaled steroid:

Beclometasone, 1 inhaler

An appropriate starting dose for most children would be 200 mcg/day. Therefore, 100 mcg twice daily in total, but often dispensed as 50 mcg metered inhalation, hence two puffs twice a day.

Potential side effects of inhaled corticosteroids are candidiasis and adrenal crisis. To reduce the risk of oral candidiasis, use a spacer device, rinse the mouth with water or brush the teeth after inhalation. Oral candidiasis should be treated with oral antifungal suspension or lozenges.

> **Role:** You are a GP
> **Setting:** GP surgery
> **Scenario:** Peter is 13 years old. He has had four episodes of complex partial seizures and an electroencephalogram (EEG) confirms the diagnosis of epilepsy. Mum is keen to commence him on medication. The paediatrician has asked you to prescribe a suitable antiepileptic medication for Peter (carbamazepine). His weight is 40 kg and height 150 cm

Carbamazepine is a drug of choice for the treatment of simple and complex partial seizures, and for tonic–clonic seizures secondary to a focal discharge:

Carbamazepine, oral
Initial dose: 5 mg/kg at night, or 2.5 mg/kg twice daily
Therefore, 5 mg/kg × 40 kg = 200 = 200 mg nocte

Carbamazepine affects the metabolism of other drugs because it is a CYP450 enzyme inducer so carbamazepine may increase the clearance of other drugs.

Other potential drug interactions include:

- Drugs that are more rapidly cleared/metabolized by carbamazepine include warfarin, theophylline, valproic acid and oral contraceptive pills.
- Drugs that reduce the metabolism of carbamazepine include cimetidine, erythromycin and calcium channel blockers.

Role: You are a GP

Setting: GP surgery

Scenario: Tara is 9 years old. She has been diagnosed with nephrotic syndrome. She is still on the initial dose of her medication. Prescribe the medication for Tara. Her weight is 25 kg and her height 135 cm

---

Prednisolone, oral
Initially 1–2 mg/kg once daily (usual maximum dose 60 mg/day)
Therefore, 1 mg/kg × 25 kg = 25 mg once daily

Information and advice to give to carer and child: indication for treatment, duration of treatment, side effects, patient information leaflet, steroid card.

Potential side effects of oral steroids include immunosuppression, adrenal suppression, mood/behaviour changes, gastrointestinal, musculoskeletal/growth and ophthalmic effects.

The cautions/contraindications are as follows: systemic infection, susceptibility to closed-angle glaucoma (including family history), osteoporosis, diabetes mellitus, hypertension, congestive heart failure.

Information on a steroid card should include the following: 1) the patient must not stop the steroids suddenly if taken for more than 3 weeks, 2) the patient must always carry the steroid card/inform healthcare professionals during and for 1 year after stopping steroids, and 3) medical attention must be sought promptly if the patient becomes unwell. The patient should avoid chicken pox if he/she has never had it before or seek urgent medical attention if he/she comes into contact with those with chicken pox.

Practice cases

- Prescribe fluids for a 6-year-old girl in an Accident and Emergency (A&E) emergency setting. Her weight is 20 kg and height 110 cm
- Prescribe a suitable antibiotic for a 7-year-old girl with a confirmed urinary tract infection (UTI). Her weight is 30 kg and height 120 cm
- Prescribe a suitable anti-epileptic medication for a 10-year-old boy with newly diagnosed tonic–clonic epilepsy. His weight is 35 kg and height 145 cm

Top tips

- Write legibly
- Remember to write the child's details (i.e. name, address) on the FP10
- Use the BNFc
- Check dosage
- Check –and then double check – your calculation

Anchor statement: safe prescribing

Station 8: Safe prescribing		
	Expected standard CLEAR PASS	PASS
PRESCRIBING EFFECTIVELY AND IN CONTEXT **(Assessment of the written prescription based on set scenario)**	Achieves both Essential and Desired criteria: **Essential:** Child's name, address, date of birth must be written on the prescription Prescribes the correct drug Writes generic drug name or trade name if appropriate Writes legibly Writes the correct dose (including zero before decimal if appropriate) and the dose strength Write dose frequency and total number of days of dose indicated Units are clearly written: g, mg, micrograms, nanograms are acceptable Completes prescription (signature, name and date of prescription) **Desired:** Checks formulations available and what would be most suitable (capsule or liquid) Dispensable dose (rounded up) Writes appropriate route of administration Fluent and confident in use of the BNFc (uses BNFc logically, acquires information rapidly, turns to appropriate pages, does not 'browse' or hunt for inspiration)	Achieves all essential criteria and some desired criteria Prescribes the correct drug OR a clinically appropriate different drug
KNOWLEDGE, SKILLS AND ATTITUDE TO PRESCRIBING **(Assessment of the discussion with the examiner)**	Explains correct choice (clinical and cost effectiveness) of medication for this scenario (based on clinical reasoning, national guideline or BNFc advice) Explains relevant patient related factors influencing prescription Knows contraindications Knows side effects Fluent and confident	Knows indications, important contraindications and side effects of the drug prescribed Aware of patient-related factors influencing prescription Lacks confidence

© Royal College of Paediatrics and Child Health 2012, reproduced with permission.

BARE FAIL	CLEAR FAIL	UNACCEPTABLE
Misses any essential criteria Prescribes the correct drug OR a clinically appropriate different drug	Misses most essential and desired criteria Prescribes the wrong drug	Unsafe prescription: · unsafe dose prescribed (correct or the wrong drug) · unsafe drug prescribed (risk to patient safety)
Limited knowledge of the drug prescribed Misses important contraindications, side effects Not aware of patient-related factors influencing prescription Lacks confidence	Limited or poor explanation offered for the choice of the drug prescribed Fails to suggest alternative and appropriate drug Poor understanding of patient-related factors influencing prescription Lacks confidence and poor responses	Lack of knowledge or understanding of contraindications, side effects Unsafe Inappropriate attitude displayed in responses

INDEX